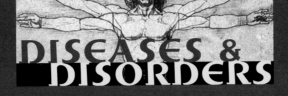

Sleep Disorders

Barbara Sheen

LUCENT BOOKS

A part of Gale, Cengage Learning

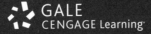

Detroit • New York • San Francisco • New Haven, Conn • Waterville, Maine • London

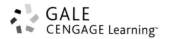

LIBRARY OF CONGRESS CATALOGING-IN-PUBLICATION DATA

Sheen, Barbara.
  Sleep disorders / by Barbara Sheen.
      pages cm. -- (Diseases & disorders)
  Includes bibliographical references and index.
  ISBN 978-1-4205-0914-4 (hardcover)
  1. Sleep disorders--Popular works. 2. Self-care, Health. I. Title.
  RC547.S473 2013
  616.8'498--dc23

                                                2012045585

Lucent Books
27500 Drake Rd.
Farmington Hills, MI 48331

ISBN-13: 978-1-4205-0914-4
ISBN-10: 1-4205-0914-4

Printed in the United States of America
1 2 3 4 5 6 7 17 16 15 14 13

Table of Contents

"The Most Difficult Puzzles Ever Devised"

Charles Best, one of the pioneers in the search for a cure for diabetes, once explained what it is about medical research that intrigued him so. "It's not just the gratification of knowing one is helping people," he confided, "although that probably is a more heroic and selfless motivation. Those feelings may enter in, but truly, what I find best is the feeling of going toe to toe with nature, of trying to solve the most difficult puzzles ever devised. The answers are there somewhere, those keys that will solve the puzzle and make the patient well. But how will those keys be found?"

Since the dawn of civilization, nothing has so puzzled people—and often frightened them, as well—as the onset of illness in a body or mind that had seemed healthy before. A seizure, the inability of a heart to pump, the sudden deterioration of muscle tone in a small child—being unable to reverse such conditions or even to understand why they occur was unspeakably frustrating to healers. Even before there were names for such conditions, even before they were understood at all, each was a reminder of how complex the human body was, and how vulnerable.

While our grappling with understanding diseases has been frustrating at times, it has also provided some of humankind's most heroic accomplishments. Alexander Fleming's accidental discovery in 1928 of a mold that could be turned into penicillin has resulted in the saving of untold millions of lives. The isolation of the enzyme insulin has reversed what was once a death sentence for anyone with diabetes. There have been great strides in combating conditions for which there is not yet a cure, too. Medicines can help AIDS patients live longer, diagnostic tools such as mammography and ultrasounds can help doctors find tumors while they are treatable, and laser surgery techniques have made the most intricate, minute operations routine.

This "toe-to-toe" competition with diseases and disorders is even more remarkable when seen in a historical continuum. An astonishing amount of progress has been made in a very short time. Just two hundred years ago, the existence of germs as a cause of some diseases was unknown. In fact, it was less than 150 years ago that a British surgeon named Joseph Lister had difficulty persuading his fellow doctors that washing their hands before delivering a baby might increase the chances of a healthy delivery (especially if they had just attended to a diseased patient)!

Each book in Lucent's Diseases and Disorders series explores a disease or disorder and the knowledge that has been accumulated (or discarded) by doctors through the years. Each book also examines the tools used for pinpointing a diagnosis, as well as the various means that are used to treat or cure a disease. Finally, new ideas are presented—techniques or medicines that may be on the horizon.

Frustration and disappointment are still part of medicine, for not every disease or condition can be cured or prevented. But the limitations of knowledge are being pushed outward constantly; the "most difficult puzzles ever devised" are finding challengers every day.

A Growing Problem

One out of every two Americans report problems falling or staying asleep. Stress, illness, a busy schedule, environmental factors, a crying infant, or a snoring mate are just a few of the things that can disturb a person's sleep. For most people, sleep disturbances occur only occasionally. But for individuals with a sleep disorder, sleep problems are ongoing and long lasting.

A sleep disorder is a condition that affects normal patterns of sleep and wakefulness. For individuals with sleep disorders, falling asleep and/or staying asleep can be torture. Some sleep too little, some too much, and some fitfully. Usually, the quality of their sleep is poor. As a result, their overall health, emotional well-being, and ability to function are compromised. British journalist Geraint Vincent knows how it feels to be sleep deprived. He spent a week during which his sleep was purposely disrupted for a television report on sleep disorders. To measure the effects of sleeplessness on daily life, he worked as a waiter during the day. "Monday was OK, I just felt a bit tired," he recalls, "but as the week wore on everything became more difficult. I really had to concentrate hard to do simple things. . . . As well as becoming phenomenally grumpy . . . my feet hurt when I walked, there was an ache in my back and I had a constant shivery feeling."[1]

A Symptom of Modern Life

Vincent was lucky; after a week he was able to return to his normal sleep pattern. But millions of people are not as fortunate. According to the American Academy of Sleep Medicine,

6

about 70 million Americans have a sleep disorder. This is more than the number of Americans with heart disease, headaches, asthma, or diabetes. Sleep disorders affect people of every age, ethnicity, and social background.

To make matters worse, the number of people with sleep disorders is growing rapidly. Although sleep disorders are not new, modern life seems to be intensifying the problem. Round-the-clock work schedules, globalization of commercial markets, stores that never close, television, and the Internet have all contributed to people's sleeping less. Americans averaged 9 hours of sleep per night in 1910. Today they average only 6.5 hours. Experts estimate that 135 million Americans voluntarily sacrifice sleep for other activities. Writer Gretchen Rubin is one of them: "Sleep feels good, so why is it so hard to turn off the light? It's because those last hours of the day are precious. TV addicts squeeze in one more show. Workaholics finish just a few more e-mails. Parents relish the peace and quiet after the kids are finally tucked into bed. Readers—and this is my temptation—want to finish just one more chapter."[2]

Although voluntary sleep deprivation may seem harmless, it is not. Over time it can disrupt healthy sleep rhythms, resulting in a sleep disorder. So, when these individuals want to get more sleep, they cannot. According to sleep expert Dr. Matthew Edlund,

> People have turned themselves into machines. They're working 24/7. But they're not machines, and their bodies aren't getting the needed rest to rebuild and renew. . . . More people are developing insomnia, so they use sleeping pills to sleep, then using stimulants like caffeine to stay awake. They race through the day, instead of going with the natural flow and rhythm. I'm saying they shouldn't fight the need to rest. The body needs time to rebuild.[3]

A Widespread Impact

Sleep disorders not only impact the individuals who suffer from them, they have a huge impact on society as a whole. This is especially true when sleep-deprived drivers get behind the

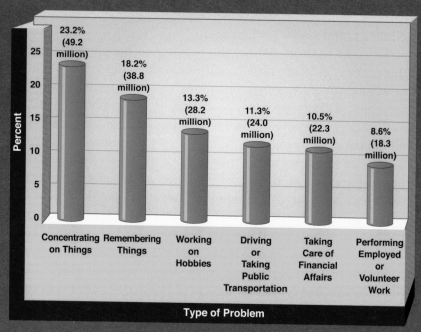

Self-Reported Sleep-Related Difficulties Among Adults Over Age Twenty, 2005–2006 and 2007–2008

Percent

- 23.2% (49.2 million) — Concentrating on Things
- 18.2% (38.8 million) — Remembering Things
- 13.3% (28.2 million) — Working on Hobbies
- 11.3% (24.0 million) — Driving or Taking Public Transportation
- 10.5% (22.3 million) — Taking Care of Financial Affairs
- 8.6% (18.3 million) — Performing Employed or Volunteer Work

Type of Problem

Taken from: Centers for Disease Control and Prevention. www.cdc.gov/features/dssleep.

wheel of a motor vehicle. When individuals do not get enough sleep, their judgment, motor skills, and alertness are impaired. They put themselves and everyone in their path at risk. According to the U.S. Department of Transportation, sleepy drivers cause about a hundred thousand car accidents a year, resulting in seventy-one thousand injuries and 1,550 deaths; that is, such drivers cause one out of every six fatal car accidents. In financial terms, this amounts to about $12.5 billion in property loss and lost productivity.

Sleep disorders also cause problems in the workplace. Individuals with sleep disorders are less productive than workers who are not sleep deprived. And sleep deprivation is the cause of many industrial accidents. Medical accidents, too, have been attributed to lack of sleep. New doctors have to work as residents in hospitals to gain experience. They typically work extended shifts without much or any sleep. A 2004 Harvard University study investigating the link between sleep deprivation and medical accidents found that 20 percent of the doctors taking part in the study reported making a fatigue-related mistake that resulted in injury to a patient. Another Harvard study examined the effect of sleep deprivation on police officers. The 2011 study screened 4,957 police officers and found that 40 percent had sleep disorders. Compared with their less-sleepy peers, sleep-deprived officers were more likely to have poorer overall health, were 22 percent more likely to be injured on the job, and were more likely to lose their tempers with suspects, which resulted in more citizen complaints against them.

The Importance of Knowledge

Clearly, sleep disorders impact everyone. Yet, many people do not understand the importance of sleep and the devastating effects of sleep deprivation. Therefore, they do not discuss their sleep problems with their doctors. An estimated 18 million Americans with sleep disorders are undiagnosed. This is particularly troubling because sleep disorders can be treated. As author D.T. Max explains:

> The social and economic costs from the undertreatment of sleeplessness are huge. The Institute of Medicine, an independent national scientific advisory group, . . . places the direct medical cost of our collective sleep debt at tens of billions of dollars. The loss in terms of work productivity is even higher. Then there are the softer costs—the damaged or lost relationships, the jobs tired people don't have the energy to apply for, the muting of enjoyment of life's pleasure. If a medical problem in some less private, less mysterious bodily function was causing such widespread harm, governments would declare war on it.[4]

The best way to solve this problem is for people to learn more about sleep and sleep disorders. Armed with knowledge, they can make lifestyle changes and seek help for themselves and their loved ones.

CHAPTER ONE

A Basic Need

A sleep disorder is a condition that disrupts normal sleeping patterns. Sleep disorders cause sleeplessness, disturbed sleep, and low-quality sleep. In order to understand sleep disorders, it is important to understand sleep.

A Mystery

Like food, water, and oxygen, all animals need sleep to survive. There is no substitute for sleep. Humans spend approximately one-third of their lives sleeping or trying to sleep. Even minimal sleep loss impacts a person's physical, mental, and emotional health. Chronic sleep deprivation is so devastating that interrogators often use it to get information from prisoners of war. When the late former Israeli prime minister Menachem Begin was held as a prisoner of war during World War II, this form of torture was used on him. He described the experience as follows: "In the head of the interrogated prisoner a haze begins to form, his spirit is wearied to death, his legs are unsteady, and he has one sole desire: to sleep. Anyone who has experienced this desire knows that not even hunger and thirst are comparable with it."[5]

Yet, despite the importance of sleep, much about it is a mystery. Scientists do not know exactly why we sleep. They do know that sleep is vital to life; that while individuals sleep, their responsiveness to outside stimuli decreases; that sleepers are easy to awaken compared with individuals in other states of reduced consciousness, such as a coma; and that all animals sleep despite the fact that sleeping makes them vulnerable to predators.

An Active Brain

Scientists also know that the brain is active during sleep. Until the 1930s, when Dr. Nathaniel Kleitman proved that the brain is active during sleep, scientists had long believed that sleep was a passive state in which the brain shuts down. Using an electroencephalograph (EEG), a device that records brain-wave patterns, Kleitman monitored and compared the brain activity

Dr. Nathaniel Kleitman's research in the 1930s proved that the brain is active during sleep, leading to further study into how sleep affects good health.

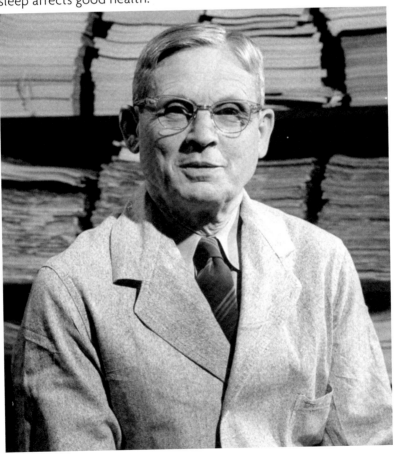

of test subjects while they were awake and while they were asleep. During an EEG, small electrodes and wires are attached to a subject's scalp. The electrodes detect electrical signals that are produced by the brain. These signals form patterns known as brain waves. The EEG machine records the brain waves as a graph on paper or on a computer screen.

Kleitman's test showed that the brain produces electrical activity during sleep as well as wakefulness. If the accepted theory that the brain shuts down during sleep were correct, then an EEG test on sleeping subjects would not have detected any activity. Although the brain-wave patterns recorded during sleep were different from those recorded during wakefulness, it was clear that the brain remained active during sleep.

Kleitman's study led to more research. Scientists now know that the brain performs a number of important jobs during sleep that are necessary to maintain good health. These include repairing, healing, and replacing damaged cells; directing the release of hormones that control growth, sexual characteristics, and appetite; restoring chemical balance; producing insulin, a hormone that turns blood sugar into energy; lowering blood pressure; strengthening the immune system; processing the experiences and emotions of the day; and creating and storing memories.

The Stages of Sleep

These functions occur during the different stages of sleep. Healthy sleep is divided into cycles. Each cycle has three initial stages followed by rapid-eye-movement, or REM, sleep. Each stage produces different brain-wave patterns, which makes it possible to recognize the stages with an EEG. The brain typically cycles through the three initial stages and REM sleep five to six times a night. A complete cycle lasts about ninety minutes, but the amount of time individuals spend in each stage of a sleep cycle changes as the sleep period progresses. Sleep disorders can interrupt, shorten, or disrupt the order of the stages or prevent one or more stages from occurring. Healthy sleep proceeds as follows.

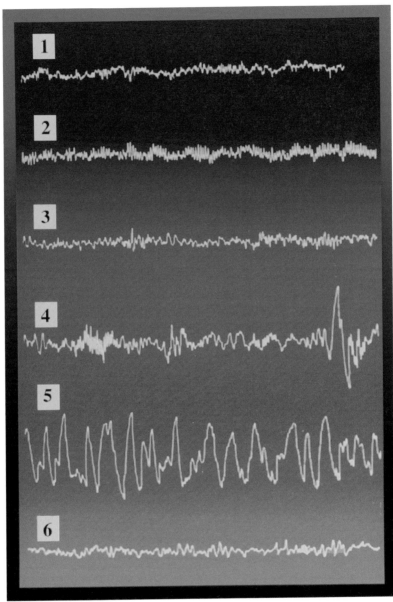

Traces from an EEG show brain waves in various states of sleep. From the top, the trace shows alpha waves of a person who is awake, followed by those of a person who is awake with eyes closed; the third and fourth traces show theta waves as a person falls asleep, with the fifth showing delta waves associated with sleep. The last trace shows brain activity during REM sleep.

Stage one is the first sleep stage. It serves as a transition between wakefulness and sleep. It constitutes 5 to 10 percent of sleep time (although, for unknown reasons, individuals with insomnia, one type of sleep disorder, may stay in stage one longer than normal). During stage one, an individual's brain and body begin to relax. Brain waves change from a combination of beta waves (rapid brain waves that dominate during wakefulness) and alpha waves (slower brain waves that occur when people are awake and relaxed) to mainly alpha waves. Breathing becomes more regular, the eyes move slowly under the eyelids, and muscle activity decreases. People often feel as if they are floating, drifting, or falling during this time. Because stage one is a very light sleep stage, sleepers can be awakened easily, and, if they are awakened, they may think that they were not asleep at all.

People at Risk

Although anyone can develop a sleep disorder, certain people are at greater risk. This group includes women experiencing hormonal changes related to menstruation, pregnancy, and menopause; people taking medications, such as stimulants, beta-blockers, steroids, and thyroid hormones; and individuals suffering from painful chronic diseases like fibromyalgia and arthritis, which makes it hard for them to get comfortable enough to fall or stay asleep.

Teenagers and young adults are another at-risk group. An estimated 7–16 percent develop circadian rhythm disorders, which sleep experts think may be linked to hormonal changes in their bodies. Shift workers whose work schedule disrupts their circadian rhythm often develop a sleep disorder, as do frequent travelers who cross multiple time zones. For unknown reasons, individuals suffering from depression and other mental disorders are also vulnerable to sleep problems.

Stage two is a deeper stage of sleep. It takes up 30 to 50 percent of sleep time. During stage two, slower, theta brain waves predominate. Sleepers' breathing and heartbeat slow and hold steady. Their eyes roll slowly under their eyelids, and, for unknown reasons, they are temporarily blind during this stage. Sleep researchers have flashed light onto the eyes of test subjects whose eyelids have been taped open during stage two sleep. The light did not disturb the sleepers, and when awakened, they did not remember seeing any light.

Stage three is the deepest stage of sleep. It is also known as slow-wave sleep (SWS) because during this stage, sleepers' brain waves slow down, and delta waves, which are the slowest of all brain waves, dominate. At this stage, sleepers' bodies are very relaxed, their body temperature is low, and their heartbeat and respiration are very slow and regular. It is difficult to wake a sleeper during stage three sleep. If individuals are awakened, they are usually quite groggy. Stage three constitutes 20 to 40 percent of sleep time.

Often people with sleep disorders do not get sufficient stage three sleep because they awaken frequently during the night. This can affect their general health, since stage three is the stage in which the brain performs much of its repair work on the body, regulates hormones, builds up energy for the next day, and strengthens memory.

REM Sleep

Stages one through three are all classified as non-rapid-eye-movement sleep stages, or nREM sleep. Shortly after stage three sleep, individuals regress to stage two sleep and then enter REM sleep. REM sleep is characterized by active eye movement in which sleepers' eyes move back and forth rapidly under closed eyelids. During REM sleep, sleepers' brain activity intensifies. Alpha and beta brain waves dominate, making the brain-wave pattern look more like that of wakefulness than of deep sleep. Sleepers' blood pressure, heart rate, and breathing rate rise, too, and dreaming occurs. And, although sleepers' small muscles may twitch, their skeletal muscles are temporarily paralyzed.

Scientists think this may be the body's way of protecting itself from physically reacting to dreams. Sleepers also dream during nREM sleep, but dreams are more concentrated in REM sleep, and REM dreams are longer and more vivid. Why people dream or what significance dreams play is another mystery. Some sleep experts think that dreaming stimulates creativity and

A colorized PET scan shows brain activity during REM sleep, with the red areas indicating areas of activity that are similar to those found when a person is awake.

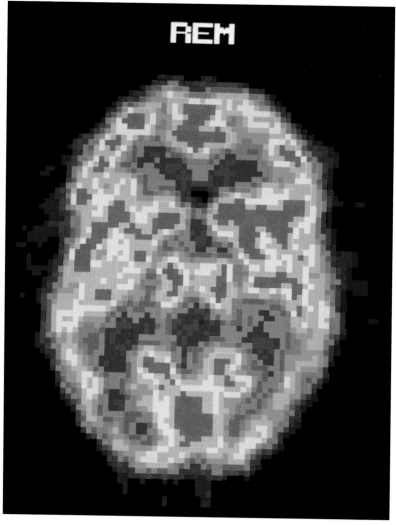

helps with problem solving, but this is not yet proven. Scientists do know that the length of dreams varies, and, when individuals are awakened from REM sleep, they usually have strong recollections of their dreams.

The exact function of REM sleep is unknown; however, sleep experts think it must be very important because if individuals are awakened at the start of a REM cycle, the next time they go to sleep they enter REM sleep more rapidly than usual, as if their bodies need to make up for the loss. One popular theory contends that during REM sleep the brain updates memories by repatterning nerve connectors in much the same manner as software defragments a computer. During this time unnecessary memories are deleted and other memories are organized.

REM sleep makes up 20 to 25 percent of sleep time. When it ends, the sleep cycle begins again. As the sleep period goes on, the duration of REM sleep increases from about ten minutes for the first episode to about one hour for the last. Conversely, nREM sleep decreases. Stage three sleep, especially, becomes briefer and briefer toward the end of the total sleep period. Since awakening from stage three sleep leaves individuals feeling groggy, shortening the duration of stage three sleep near the time of awakening may be the brain's way of making sure individuals wake up feeling refreshed.

Sleeping and Waking

Exactly when individuals fall asleep and when they wake up is controlled by two important mechanisms called homeostasis and circadian rhythms. Homeostasis keeps the body in balance so that it can function correctly. Among other things, homeostasis drives the body to sleep when it is tired. As sleep disorder expert Dr. Nancy Foldvary-Schaefer explains: "Bodies naturally maintain an internal equilibrium; this is called homeostasis. Just as our stomach growls when we feel hunger pangs, and our throat is dry when we are thirsty . . . we have a homeostatic drive to sleep. Our brain tells us when it's time for lights out."[6]

The brain also regulates the body's circadian rhythm, its daily internal clock, which works with homeostasis and with the external environment to coordinate sleep and wakefulness. The body's circadian clock is like an alarm clock in the brain that is controlled by light and darkness. Darkness signals the clock that it is time to sleep, which causes the brain to release melatonin, a chemical that makes individuals feel sleepy. Light coming in through the eyelids suppresses the release of melatonin and signals the clock that it is time to wake up. In some sleep disorders, the circadian clock may be disturbed, delaying the release of melatonin. The release of melatonin can also be disrupted if individuals are deprived of sunlight during the day or exposed to excessive light at night.

How Much Sleep Is Enough?

Not everybody needs the same amount of sleep. The amount of sleep people require depends on a number of factors. Age is one of the most important. On average, adults need 8 hours of sleep per night to maintain good health. Teenagers need 9 hours. School-age children need 9 to 10 hours, whereas children aged one to five need 11 to 13 hours, and infants about 16 hours. Sick people of any age require extra sleep, as do pregnant women in the first trimester (the first three months) of pregnancy.

The amount of sleep individuals need also increases if they did not get enough sleep the night before. This is known as sleep debt. Sleep debt is the difference between the amount of sleep individuals need and the amount of sleep they get. Every time individuals sleep less than they should, they add to their sleep debt. People with sleep disorders usually have very large sleep debts.

Like financial debt, sleep debt should be paid back. Many people try to pay back their sleep debt by sleeping longer on the weekend or on their days off work or school. But a few hours of extra sleep on Saturday cannot pay back the sleep debt of individuals who are chronically sleep deprived. For instance, if individuals sleep three hours less than they need per night, in a week they have accrued 21 hours of sleep debt; in a month, 84 hours; and in a year, 1,008 hours. "It starts out

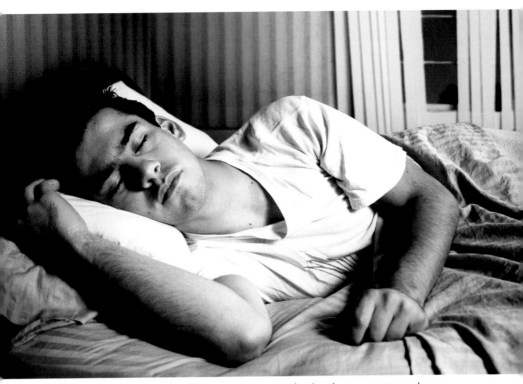

The darkness of nighttime prompts the body to want to sleep because of circadian rhythms, which also regulate wakefulness as a response to light.

small," explains sleep expert Michael Breus, "but the effects compound quickly. Let it go too long and you may never be able to pay it all back."[7]

Eventually, the brain will insist that sleep debt be paid off. Coming down with a cold or flu, which causes patients to stay in bed and sleep, is one way the body may try to catch up. If one's sleep debt is too large, however, it may be impossible to ever pay it all back. And, because lack of sleep negatively affects a person's mental and physical well-being, sleep debt detracts from a person's waking life. A 2010 Australian study found that an individual's risk of feeling depressed, stressed, or anxious increases by 14 percent for every hour of missed sleep. This is not surprising since lack of sleep increases levels of cortisol, a hormone linked to stress.

American Sleep Habits

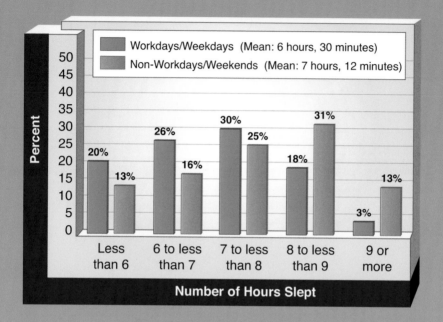

All respondents were asked how long they typically sleep on both a typical workday or weekday and a typical non-workday or weekend.

Overall, respondents reported that they typically sleep less on workdays or weekdays than on non-workdays or weekends (6 hours and 30 minutes v. 7 hours and 12 minutes, on average).

- In fact, the proportion who slept at least 8 hours on non-workdays or weekends is more than twice the proportion who do so on weekdays or workdays (44 percent v. 21 percent).

- Notably, those who say they get a good night's sleep every day or almost every day get about an hour more of sleep on workdays or weekdays (7 hours 9 minutes v. 6 hours 2 minutes) and on non-workdays or weekends (7 hours 41 minutes v. 6 hours and 52 minutes) on average compared to their counterparts.

Bodily Effects of Sleep Debt

Even a small sleep debt can affect a person's health. For people with sleep disorders who have large sleep debts, the effects on the body can be overwhelming. Sleep deprivation has been linked to heart disease, high blood pressure, obesity, diabetes, headaches, backaches, general pain, memory loss, and shortened attention span. A 2008 University of Chicago study found that for unknown reasons, lack of sleep increases the buildup of plaque, a form of hardened fats, calcium, and other material in the arteries. Plaque is dangerous because it can break off and block smaller blood vessels, causing a heart attack or stroke. The researchers looked at 495 men and women aged thirty-five to forty-seven. They found that 27 percent of the subjects that averaged five hours of sleep per night had plaque in their coronary arteries (the arteries of the heart itself), compared with just 6 percent of those who slept more than seven hours per night.

Another University of Chicago study, conducted in 2012, also found a strong link between sleep deprivation and heart disease. In this study, researchers looked at 3,019 subjects aged forty-five or older who were participating in a survey aimed at assessing a variety of health issues. The study showed that people getting less than six hours of sleep each night were 2 times more likely to have a stroke or heart attack and 1.6 times more likely to have congestive heart failure than were the participants who got seven or eight hours of sleep. According to Dr. Tracy Stevens of the American Heart Association, "We have enough evidence from this study and others to show that it is important to include sleep in any discussion of heart disease. We talk about the traditional risk factors, and now the other important thing we need to include is sleep."[8]

Diabetes

Diabetes, a disease that affects the body's ability to convert glucose, or blood sugar, to energy and that can lead to kidney failure and blindness, has also been linked to sleep deprivation. In fact, a number of studies have shown that sleeping four hours or less for as little as two nights can affect the body's ability to produce insulin, a hormone that regulates blood glucose levels. Once individuals get adequate sleep, insulin production returns to normal. If sleep deprivation becomes chronic, however, insulin production stays disrupted, and blood sugar levels can rise to abnormal levels, putting people at risk of developing diabetes.

Diabetes is also associated with obesity, and lack of sleep has been shown to lead to weight gain. Sleep deprivation lowers the production of an appetite-suppressing hormone known as leptin while boosting an appetite-inducing hormone known as ghrelin. As a result, sleep-deprived individuals eat more than well-rested individuals. A 2011 study at New York's Columbia University, showed that subjects who slept for four hours a night for six nights ate three hundred more calories per day than did subjects who slept for nine hours. The study also found that the sleep-deprived subjects craved calorie-laden junk food. A 2007 University of Chicago study had almost identical findings. According to Chicago researcher Eve Van Cauter,

> Subjects who had the most disrupted levels of leptin and ghrelin were the ones who felt the hungriest. Their appetite for cakes, candy, ice cream, potato chips, pasta and bread increased, though their appetite for fruits, vegetables, and high-protein nutrients did not. We don't know why food choice would shift, but since the brain is fueled by glucose, we suspect it seeks simple carbohydrates when distressed by lack of sleep.[9]

To make matters worse, lack of sleep leaves people too tired to work off the extra calories they consume, and, according to a 2011 study at Sweden's Uppsala University, sleep deprivation slows down individuals' waking metabolism, which means they burn fewer calories.

Obesity

On the basis of these findings, it is not surprising to learn that a number of other studies have shown that sleep deprivation

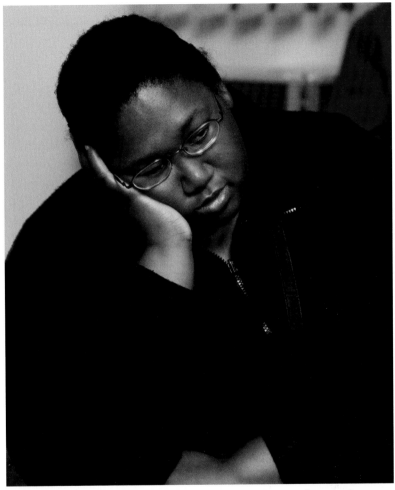

Sleep deprivation can have more serious effects than making a person tired during the day. It has also been linked to heart disease, high blood pressure, obesity, diabetes, memory loss, and other serious health conditions.

is associated with obesity. For instance, a Columbia University study that tracked 6,115 adults found that subjects who slept an average of four hours per night were 73 percent more likely to be obese than those who slept seven to nine hours. More than thirty-one other studies have found a strong connection between short sleep duration in children and future obesity. Interestingly, in the last fifty years, the incidence of obesity

How Animals Sleep

Sleep is essential to all animals. Some animals have unique ways of sleeping, which help them guard against predators and other dangers while asleep. A walrus, for example, is an aquatic mammal that needs air. Before going to sleep, it inflates pouches inside its body with air. The pouches act like a life jacket, allowing the walrus to sleep in a vertical position while keeping its head above water. A sea otter, another aquatic mammal, sleeps floating on its back wrapped in seaweed. The seaweed acts like an anchor, keeping the otter from floating out to sea. Mallard ducks also sleep floating on the water. They sleep in a line. The two outermost birds sleep with one eye open and part of their brain alert, so they can watch for predators.

Horses often lie down to sleep. They can also sleep standing up, with their legs locked to maintain their balance. Sleeping upright lets horses escape from predators quickly. Squirrels protect themselves from predators by sleeping in nests high up in trees. In cold weather, squirrels sleep huddled together in the nest to keep warm.

Two otters stay afloat in the sea while sleeping on their backs.

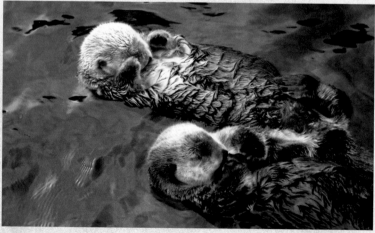

has more than doubled in the United States while sleep time has also been reduced. Some sleep researchers think there is a direct correlation.

Compromised Immunity

Lack of sleep also compromises the immune system. A number of studies have shown that sleep deprivation reduces the production of infection-fighting T-cells, making it more difficult for individuals to fight off infections. A 2009 study at Carnegie Mellon University in Pittsburgh found that healthy test subjects who slept less than seven hours per night were almost three times more likely to become sick after being exposed to a cold virus than were subjects who slept eight hours per night.

These health issues are just the tip of the iceberg. Lack of sleep has also been linked to colon cancer, memory loss, reduced cognitive abilities, dementia, attention-deficit/hyperactivity disorder, and mental illnesses, among other conditions. Author Gayle Greene, who suffers from insomnia, has direct experience with the effects of sleep deprivation:

> My body tells me things are not right when I lose sleep, and they're not right all the way through: my heart is working overtime, I'm metabolically deranged, cold all the time, hollow at the core. I eat like I'm stoking a dying fire, not for the pleasure but for the energy, and my mood hits the wall. . . . If I get on a plane or swim too long I get a cold. My body needles me with a whole host of ailments— arthritis, gum disease, autoimmune problems, persistent rashes, allergies.[10]

Without a doubt, lack of sleep is dangerous to an individual's health. Although many aspects of sleep remain a mystery, it is clear that sleep is a basic need. Consequently, people with sleep disorders face multiple health threats. Since there are many different kinds of sleep disorders, in order to treat them, it is important to distinguish between these different kinds.

CHAPTER TWO

Many Disorders

Scientists have identified more than eighty different sleep disorders. To make understanding sleep disorders easier, they are classified into six categories: insomnia, sleep-related breathing disorders, sleep-related movement disorders, parasomnias, circadian rhythm disorders, and hypersomnias.

Insomnia

Insomnia is the most common of all sleep disorders. People with insomnia have problems falling asleep, staying asleep, and/or awakening too early. Insomnia can be temporary, lasting from a day to a month. This type of insomnia is usually caused by excitement or worry before a major event in a person's life, a temporary illness that disrupts sleep, or a single ongoing stressful situation. But once the illness, worry, stress, or excitement passes, individuals quickly revert to normal sleep patterns.

Insomnia that occurs on most nights for at least a month is known as chronic insomnia. Chronic insomnia can plague people for much of their lives. As one middle-aged insomniac explains: "I can't remember ever being able to sleep! . . . As a child I remember being the only one awake at slumber parties. I don't know how I made it in college on such little sleep."[11]

One out of five individuals suffers from chronic insomnia. In many cases, chronic insomnia arises as a symptom of another sleep disorder or long-term health problem that interferes with sleep, or as a side effect of medications that suppress sleep.

This is known as secondary insomnia. Most cases of chronic insomnia, however, are not linked to other conditions. These cases are known as primary insomnia.

Experts do not know what causes primary insomnia. Some cases seem to run in families, but a gene linked to the condition has not yet been identified. Other cases are associated with poor sleep habits and/or chronic anxiety and stress. In many instances the cause cannot be explained. According to Daniel Buysee of the University of Pittsburgh School of Medicine, "We do not know the real cause of insomnia. . . . We do not know the nature of the basic neural mechanisms [brain activity] underlying primary insomnia. . . . The genetics of the disorder are also unknown."[12]

Insomnia can occur at the onset of sleep. This is known as sleep onset insomnia. Although most people fall asleep in about ten minutes, it can take hours for people with sleep onset insomnia to fall asleep. Many people with sleep onset

One in five people suffers from chronic insomnia, which causes problems with falling asleep or staying asleep.

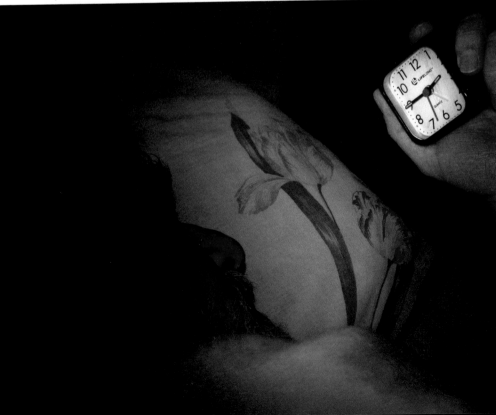

insomnia say they have trouble turning off their minds. As soon as they shut their eyes, they are plagued by feelings of anxiety, including anxiety about not being able to fall asleep. As one insomniac explains, "Just the thought of going to bed starts the anxiety all over again. Clock-watching is my night, struggling to stay awake is my day. Why can't I turn off my brain when I go to bed?"[13] Sleep onset insomniacs tend to spend more time in less-refreshing stage one sleep than do other sleepers. Many misinterpret the light sleep of stage one sleep for wakefulness, thinking that they have not slept when they actually have.

Some insomniacs wake up frequently during the night and find it difficult to fall back to sleep. Since repeated awakenings disrupt normal sleep cycles, these individuals do not get good-quality sleep. Award-winning actor George Clooney is among this group. "I have a very tough time getting to sleep," he admits. "Without question I wake every night five times."[14]

Other insomniacs sleep well until about 3 A.M., when they awaken and are unable to get back to sleep. Since rapid-eye-movement, or REM, sleep increases as the night goes on, this type of insomnia reduces REM sleep. Interestingly, besides feeling the effects of sleep deprivation the next day, many of these individuals report problems with their memory. Because sleep patterns seem to change as individuals age, elderly people often have this type of insomnia. And, for unknown reasons, so do people suffering from depression.

Sleep-Related Breathing Disorders

People with sleep-related breathing disorders experience pauses in their breathing during sleep, causing reduced oxygen levels in the blood. Sleep-related breathing disorders are almost as common as insomnia. Indeed, the most common sleep-related breathing disorder—obstructive sleep apnea (the medical term for not breathing)—is also the second most common sleep disorder. It affects more than 18 million Americans.

There are two types of sleep apnea, obstructive and central sleep apnea. In central sleep apnea, the brain fails to control breathing during sleep. Central sleep apnea is rare. Generally,

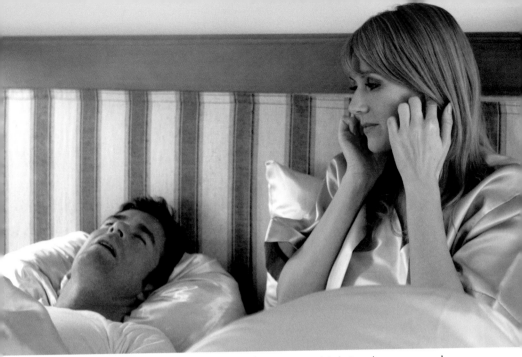

Sleep apnea can result in loud snoring, which is why a person's bed partner is usually the first to notice a sleep-related breathing disorder.

when medical professionals talk about sleep apnea, they are talking about obstructive sleep apnea, which is caused by a blockage, or obstruction, of the airway in the throat. Muscles throughout the body relax during sleep. In people with obstructive sleep apnea, the throat muscles become so relaxed that they collapse and temporarily block the flow of air in and out of the lungs.

People with sleep apnea stop breathing for intervals of ten seconds to two minutes while they are asleep. This causes them to wake up for a few seconds to catch their breath. These episodes can occur hundreds of times a night. Although some individuals have trouble going back to sleep, most usually fall back to sleep without being aware of what happened. Frequent awakenings, however, cause individuals with sleep apnea to spend more time in stage one sleep than is normal and less time in the more restorative stage three. This is one reason why they feel very tired the next day. In fact, many people with sleep apnea report falling asleep at inappropriate times during the day. Mike, who was recently diagnosed with sleep apnea, recalls,

For years I had been getting sleepier and sleepier. I went to bed early, but woke up the next morning feeling dragged out and unrested. I used to sit on the edge of the bed in the morning and count the hours till I could take a nap. I fell asleep at work, and I am a teacher. I had 32 beady little pairs of eyes just waiting for me to nod off! I fell asleep during the 5 o'clock news. I dragged off to bed at 8:30 or 9:00 at night and woke up the next morning to start the whole thing all over.[15]

Often sleep apnea patients' bed partners are the first to suspect a problem. As sleepers struggle to breathe, they produce extremely loud snores, followed by silence when they stop breathing, and then a gasp for air. Snoring associated with sleep apnea is much louder than the snores of healthy sleepers. Normal snoring

Jet Lag

Jet lag is a feeling of extreme fatigue that occurs when people cross multiple time zones in rapid succession. It is a circadian rhythm disorder in which a traveler's circadian clock functions on the light-dark sleep time of their place of origin, rather than on that of the place they traveled to. This puts them out of sync with the local time. For instance, a traveler going from New York to London crosses five time zones. If the traveler leaves New York at 5 P.M. and arrives in London seven hours later, the traveler's circadian clock, which is on New York time, thinks it is 12 A.M., time for bed, but the time in London, however, is 5 A.M., nearly time to wake up and start the day.

Symptoms of jet lag include sleepiness, headaches, insomnia, memory problems, digestive upsets, and irritability. Jet lag is a temporary condition that rectifies as the brain gradually adjusts its circadian clock to the new time by an hour or two a day. Therefore, it takes three to five days for a New York-to-London traveler's circadian clock to readjust.

is about 60 to 70 decibels loud. Snoring associated with sleep apnea measures about 90 decibels, equivalent to a lawn mower or a chain saw. Often, this nighttime noise awakens family members who alert the sleeper to the problem. It was Mike's wife who sent him to a sleep doctor: "My wife said not only did I snore like a hog, I choked, gasped, snorted and gurgled, and then would suddenly quit it all until I started again with a choking gasp."[16]

Certain physical characteristics are associated with sleep apnea. These include crowded airways caused by enlarged tonsils or adenoids (tissue between the back of the nose and throat), a large tongue, a wide neck, and/or obesity. Excess weight can produce extra fat in the neck, which contributes to an airway blockage. It also puts pressure on the airways, reducing individuals' ability to take breaths during sleep. Ironically, since sleep apnea disrupts stage three sleep, which is the part of sleep in which appetite-controlling hormones are regulated, individuals with sleep apnea tend to gain weight, which worsens the condition. And, although people with sleep apnea are not likely to suffocate, apnea episodes can cause blood oxygen levels to fall dangerously low. This causes the heart to work harder and raises blood pressure, putting individuals at risk of heart attack and stroke.

Sleep-Related Movement Disorders

Other sleep disorders involve simple involuntary movements that make it difficult for individuals to fall and stay asleep. Restless legs syndrome is the most common. People with restless legs syndrome complain of mild to severe tingling, burning, and aching in their legs, which usually begins at night and ends in the morning. The feeling can only be relieved by getting up and moving the legs. Relief, however, is temporary, and individuals with restless legs syndrome spend much of each night pacing the floor. As a result, they are sleep deprived, and what sleep they do get is poor quality. Thomas Perkins, a neurologist in Raleigh, North Carolina, describes the feeling as "a creepy-crawly sensation that occurs deep inside, near the bone, so you can't scratch it away or change positions the way you could if you had a muscle cramp or a compressed nerve."[17]

In 2007 scientists at Emory University in Atlanta identified a gene that makes individuals susceptible to developing restless legs syndrome. But genetics does not appear to be the only cause. Up to 25 percent of pregnant women develop the condition during pregnancy, but the symptoms usually disappear after they give birth. Some cases seem to be linked to anemia,

People with restless legs syndrome have their sleep disrupted by pain and tingling that is only relieved when they move their legs.

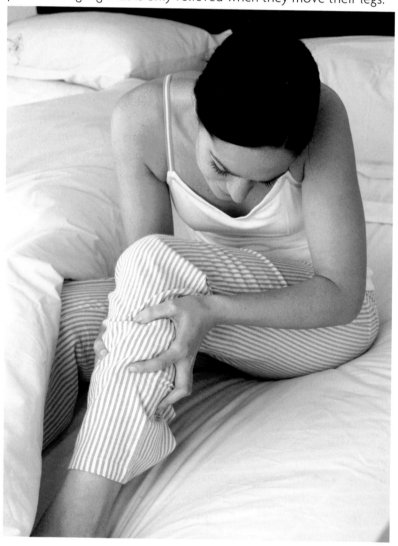

a medical condition characterized by an iron deficiency. Scientists theorize that lack of iron causes brain signals to misfire, resulting in the symptoms of restless legs syndrome.

Sleepwalking, Talking, and Other Activities

Sleep disorders known as parasomnias also involve movement. Individuals with a parasomnia perform involuntary physical activities that range from sitting up in bed looking confused to walking, talking, eating, screaming, head banging, and teeth grinding while asleep. All parasomnias disrupt sleep and normal sleep cycles.

Experts do not know what causes parasomnias. They believe something goes wrong in the sleeper's brain as it moves in or out of stage three sleep, causing part of the brain to become partially awake while another part is in deep sleep. This puts sleepers in a "twilight" world where they are not fully awake nor fully asleep. It allows them to perform physical activities associated with wakefulness that they do not remember doing upon awakening.

It is difficult to awaken sleepers during a parasomnia episode. If sleepers are awakened, they are likely to be confused. Both adults and children suffer from parasomnias, but certain types of parasomnia, such as night terrors, occur predominantly in children. Persons having night terrors exhibit signs of panic while sleeping; their hearts pound; their breathing accelerates; they scream in fear and sweat profusely. An episode lasts from five to forty-five minutes. When it is over, the victim sleeps calmly as if nothing happened. Author Laura Linley describes how night terrors affected her daughter: "She would wake nightly . . . with a piercing cry and was inconsolable for a good 10 minutes. After the arousal ran its course she would then silently sleep."[18]

Rhythmic movement disorder, which is characterized by episodes of head banging, head rolling, and/or body rocking during sleep, is another parasomnia that mainly affects children. So is confusional arousal, a condition in which sleepers sit up in bed with their eyes open, appear confused, then fall back into a normal sleep state.

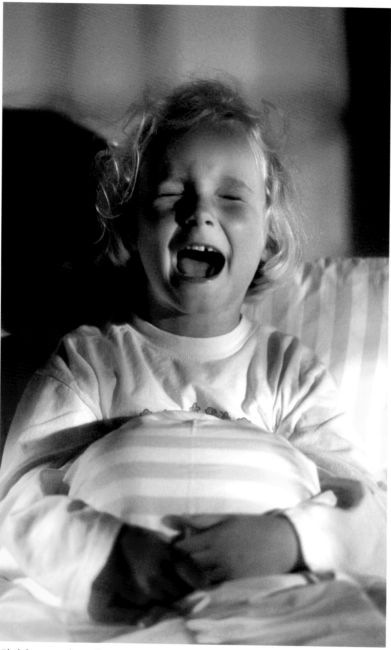

Children with night terrors experience episodes of panic and screaming during sleep that they do not remember when they awake.

Other types of parasomnias affect individuals of all ages. Some, like sleep talking, a condition in which individuals unknowingly talk, mumble, or sing in their sleep, do not pose a danger to the sleeper. Others, like teeth grinding, or bruxism, a condition in which people grind their teeth and clench their jaws while asleep, pose a greater risk. Individuals with bruxism can ruin their teeth and, in severe cases, break their jawbone. Episodes of teeth grinding can be brief or can last for hours, depending on the individual.

Sleepwalking puts individuals in perhaps the greatest peril. The majority of sleepwalkers are children, but 5 to 7 percent of adults sleepwalk, too. Sleepwalking episodes last from five to fifteen minutes and usually occur one or two times per month, although some sleepwalkers have episodes every night. At first glance, sleepwalkers appear to be awake. Their eyes are open and they may babble incoherently. But they have no awareness or control over their activities. They have only limited awareness of their environment, and their coordination and judgment are poor. Sleepwalkers have been known to urinate in inappropriate places, wander aimlessly outdoors, light fires, drive a car, and fall out of a window. As one sleepwalker explains: "My mom told me during one of my sleepwalks to move my car, she obviously didn't know I was sleepwalking. I went out and moved the car and don't remember doing it. . . . Very scary!!!"[19]

Some sleepwalkers may prepare food and eat during a sleepwalking episode. These individuals can cut or burn themselves while trying to "cook" and face the risk of choking. Also, they have been known to eat inappropriate items such as pet food, ashes, and soap. As with all parasomnias, these individuals have no memory of their behavior. As one woman explains:

> I kept blaming my kids and my husband for messing up the kitchen when I went to bed at night. Finally after months of this, I set up a video camera to catch the midnight eater. It only took a few nights to see that it was me! How could I walk through my house, make a mess in my kitchen, eat, and not remember a thing, or wake up? No wonder I was gaining weight![20]

Mixing Up Night and Day

Circadian rhythm disorders are another form of sleep disorder. These disorders are caused by a misalignment between the body's circadian clock and the external environment. Delayed sleep phase syndrome is among the most common circadian rhythm disorders. In this disorder, individuals' circadian clocks run behind that of the external environment. People with this disorder do not feel sleepy until 1 A.M. or later, instead of a more normal time, like 10 P.M. Some do not feel sleepy until dawn. They therefore have trouble waking up in the morning and functioning on a normal schedule. And, since their sleep period is shortened, they get less REM sleep than they need. Psychologist John Cline describes how delayed sleep phase syndrome affects a teenager named Kristen:

> She doesn't go to bed until 3 A.M. This is not because she has a hard time falling asleep once she gets in bed. She does not have insomnia. She only has trouble falling asleep if she goes to bed before 3 A.M. At 3 A.M. she is able to easily fall asleep. She does not find it easy, however, to get up at 6:30 A.M., which is the last possible time she can get up and still make it to school on time. In fact, her mother and father practically have to pull her out of bed to get her up. When she does make it to school on time, she often falls asleep during her morning classes. . . . She is tired all the time and can be irritable. Her grades have suffered as well.[21]

Delayed sleep phase syndrome can be caused by a defect in the body's circadian clock. But most cases are caused by people voluntarily staying up late, night after night, until this behavior causes their circadian clock to reset. Interestingly, about 5 to 10 percent of teenagers have delayed sleep phase syndrome. During puberty hormonal changes in a teen's body cause their circadian rhythm to shift slightly, resulting in delays in the time they are ready to go to bed and the time they are ready to wake up. Scientists think an unknown gene may cause this shift to be more severe in some teens. The shift usually normalizes as

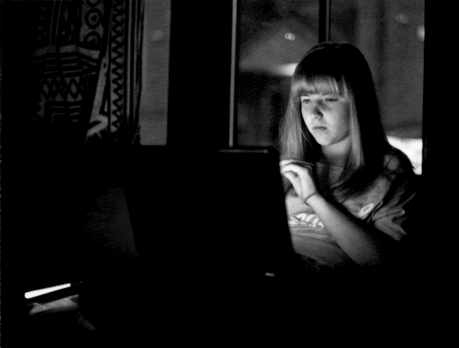

Teenagers who stay up late using computers, televisions, and other devices can have a hard time falling asleep. The devices emit bright light that can cause their circadian clock to reset.

teens become adults and hormone levels stabilize. What makes matters worse is that many teens stay up late using computers, playing video games, texting, and watching television. These activities expose users to bright light, which causes the body to suppress the release of melatonin. Over time, this behavior can delay the circadian clock even further.

Uncontrollable Sleep

Sleep disorders known as hypersomnias cause excessive daytime sleepiness. Narcolepsy is the most common. It affects one in two thousand Americans. In the past, medical professionals believed that narcolepsy was a form of mental illness. They now think it is a physical disorder caused by an abnormality in the brain that affects the transmission of hypocretin, a chemical that helps regulate sleep.

People with narcolepsy have uncontrollable attacks of daytime sleepiness that make them fall asleep at inappropriate times. Sleep attacks can last from a few seconds to several minutes and can occur multiple times throughout the day

Sleep and Athletic Performance

One of the safest and easiest ways for athletes to get an edge on their competition is to get more sleep. A 2011 Stanford University study looked at the effect of increased sleep on the school's basketball team. Team members were asked to sleep normally for two to four weeks. Most slept an average of 6.7 hours per night. At the end of this time, the team members' shooting percentages from various distances and their running speed were measured. Then, the team members were asked to spend 10 hours a night in bed for the next five to seven weeks. Although most of the athletes did not sleep for the full 10 hours, most averaged 8.5 hours a night, an increase of about 111 minutes. At the end of the study the subjects' athletic performance was measured again. With more sleep, their shooting percentages increased by about 9 percent, and their running speed improved by about 4 percent. A comparable 2008 Stanford University study focusing on the swim team yielded similar performance improvements.

without warning. As Stephanie Handy, a twenty-five-year-old woman with narcolepsy, explains:

> During a sleep attack I find that my eyes will not stay open. . . . As sleep comes, suddenly I can feel my neck and head slump onto my shoulder. My arms are relaxed and weakened. I may attempt to sit or 'fall' into the chair, sometimes injuring myself when sitting or laying down since I have decreased ability to control my descent. These attacks cause me a lot of grief. . . . I've had them at concerts, movies, watching TV, playing video games and even while reading books. I don't know of any activity I've done that hasn't been interrupted by a sleep attack at some time in my life.[22]

Narcolepsy also affects nightly sleep. When people with narcolepsy go to sleep at night, rather than going through a normal sleep cycle, they immediately fall into REM sleep. This disruption in their sleep cycle decreases the quality of their sleep and causes them to wake frequently during the night. Since they skip the initial stages of sleep and begin their sleep in REM, their brains do not shift fully into sleep mode. As a result, during the time that narcoleptics shift from wakefulness to sleep and vice versa, their dreams often seem like they are actually happening, much like a hallucination. They may also be aware of the paralysis that accompanies REM sleep, which can make the whole experience even more frightening.

For unknown reasons, some people with narcolepsy are subjected to this temporary paralysis while they are fully

People with narcolepsy fall asleep during the day at inappropriate times, but often have trouble staying asleep at night.

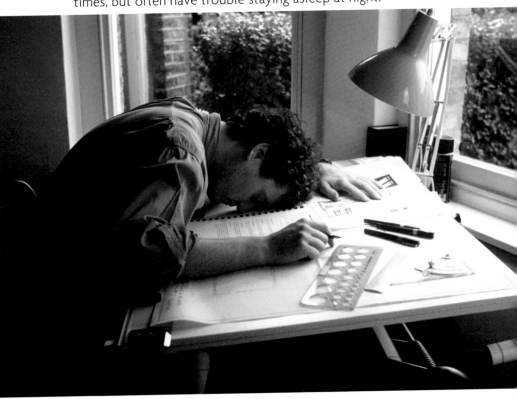

conscious. This is known as cataplexy. "Imagine a puppet on strings and suddenly the strings, which are your muscle tone, are immediately let go and so you fall to the ground,"[23] explains Bob Cloud, a patient with cataplexy.

Cataplexy is triggered by emotions such as fear, laughter, or anger and parallels the temporary paralysis of the skeletal muscles that occurs during REM sleep. Attacks are unpredictable and can occur dozens of times in a given week and rarely the next. Whenever the attacks occur, they put people at risk of serious injury. Handy recalls an injurious attack: "I was happily roller skating near my house when my knees suddenly buckled. . . . When I hit the ground, I fractured my wrist. Fully conscious, I was unable to do anything."[24]

Clearly, sleep disorders cause many problems. The first step in dealing with these problems is getting an accurate diagnosis so that treatment can begin.

CHAPTER THREE

Diagnosis and Treatment

Diagnosing sleep disorders often requires patients to spend a night at a sleep center, where health care professionals record and monitor their brain waves and bodily functions as they sleep. Treatment depends on the individual and the specific sleep disorder. It may involve the use of special devices, sleep medication, and/or behavioral therapy. Some patients turn to less traditional treatments.

The First Step

When sleep problems affect a person's daily life, it is time to see a sleep specialist, a physician who specializes in treating sleep disorders. Before the visit, patients are usually asked to record information about their sleep history in a sleep log. This information helps physicians better understand the patients' sleep troubles.

During the initial visit, the doctor checks for illnesses that can cause secondary insomnia and examines the patient's airways and mouth for signs of enlarged tonsils, adenoids, or tongue, which can cause sleep apnea. The doctor questions the patient about any emotional problems that might be affecting sleep. If a sleep disorder is suspected, the patient is usually asked to spend the night at a sleep center.

Visiting a Sleep Center

A sleep center is a medical center where patients sleep hooked up to equipment used to diagnose sleep disorders. Rooms in a sleep center resemble a hotel suite. After the patient dresses in sleepwear and gets into bed, a sleep technician tapes electrodes to the patient's head, near the eyes, nose, and mouth, as well as to the chest, chin, and legs. This is painless. The sensors are connected by nonrestricting wires to a polysomnograph, a machine that includes an electroencephalograph (EEG) as well as other devices that measure muscle activity, airflow from the mouth and nose, blood oxygen levels, and heartbeat. A computer converts the information into graphs, which tell when and how long the patient slept, how often and for how long the patient awakened during the night, when the patient entered the different stages of sleep, when and if the patient stopped breathing, and how long it took for the patient to resume breathing. A video camera and speakers record any movements or sounds the sleeping patient makes. Sleep technicians monitor the patient and the equipment.

The accommodations are designed to encourage sleep. The bed is comfortable, and the room is kept cool, quiet, and dark. Still, the sensors, the stress of being watched by strangers, and the unfamiliar bed and surroundings make it difficult for some patients to fall asleep. When this occurs, patients are administered a sleeping pill. Yet, many patients fall asleep more easily than they expect to. New York attorney Eric Fields describes his experience:

> The day of the study, I felt anxious about sleeping in front of a video camera, but I showed up for my 10 P.M. appointment, answered a sleep-habit questionnaire, and entered my room. It looked like a simple three-star hotel room. . . . Technicians attached electrodes . . . to my chest, head, and ankles to measure my heart rate, breathing, brain activity, and eye and leg movements. Equipment ran up and down my body, and multicolored wires dangled from my head, making me feel like a lab rat. . . . Although the wires were a bit uncomfortable, I drifted off to sleep easier than expected.[25]

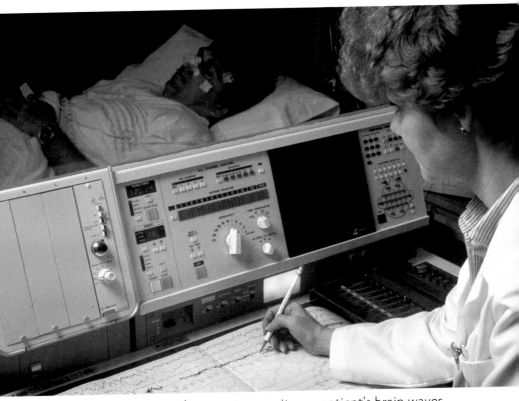

A technician at a sleep center monitors a patient's brain waves, heart rate, breathing, and muscle activity to determine the nature of his sleep disorder.

Patients are awakened by the technicians in the morning. Those who appear to have narcolepsy are asked to return to the sleep center during the day to assess their daytime sleep episodes.

Evaluating the Results

After the sleep study, technicians score the results of the polysomnogram, using numbers and percentages. The information is divided into a number of categories, including time in bed; total sleep time; sleep time spent in each stage of sleep; sleep latency, or the time it takes the patient to fall asleep; rapid-eye-movement (REM) latency, or the time from sleep onset to the first start of REM; number of apnea episodes per hour; blood oxygen levels; and the number of periodic limb movements that awaken the patient. The technician also reviews the video and audio recordings, noting any abnormalities, such as what sleep position patients are in when apnea episodes occur. The sleep specialist uses the scoring and the technician's notes to make a diagnosis. Once this is done, treatment can begin.

Sleeping with a Mask

Treatment for sleep disorders depends on the specific disorder and the individual. For instance, in cases of sleep apnea, overweight patients are advised to lose weight since excess fat in the neck can impair breathing. And, if apnea episodes occur mainly while patients sleep on their backs, patients are told to avoid sleeping in this position.

Back sleeping is a problem for many people with sleep apnea. It causes the tongue to flop backward, which can block the airway. To keep from sleeping on their backs, some patients wear a tight-fitting sleep shirt with a tennis ball stuffed in the back, which makes it uncomfortable to sleep on their backs.

People with sleep apnea are also treated with positive airway pressure (PAP) therapy. PAP therapy utilizes a small air-blowing machine connected to a special mask, which sleepers wear over their noses or over both their mouths and noses. The air flow forces the sleeper's airway to stay open during the night, reducing sleep apnea episodes. Air flow pressure is based on each patient's individual needs. In general, more severe cases need stronger air pressure than do milder cases.

There are several different types of PAP therapy. Continuous positive airway pressure (CPAP) and bilevel positive airway pressure (bi-PAP) are the most common. In CPAP therapy, the pressure of the air delivered to the mask is continuous. In bi-PAP, the pressure decreases slightly when the patient exhales, which makes it easier for some individuals to breathe. As Tracy, a sleep apnea patient, explains: "I spent the better part of the first year after diagnosis on CPAP. I was never able to tolerate it completely. . . . [It] left me feeling a sensation of suffocation and choking. I was never able to keep the mask on for more than a few hours per night . . . [but] I was immediately able to tolerate BiLevel and experienced the first good sleep I had had in probably ten or fifteen years."[26]

PAP therapy masks also vary. Some only cover the nostrils, while others cover the mouth and nose. Doctors work with

A man gets relief from his sleep apnea symptoms by wearing a CPAP machine, which uses air pressure to force open the airways in his mouth and nose while he is sleeping.

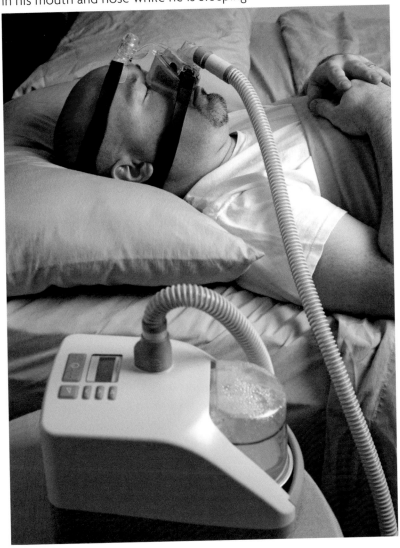

A Controversial Treatment

A drug called gamma hydroxybutyrate (GHB) has been found to be an effective treatment for narcolepsy and cataplexy. When it is taken at night, it produces extreme sleepiness and normalizes sleep cycles. It also reduces daytime sleepiness and cataplexy episodes by 85 percent, even in cases where no other treatment works. GHB, however, is a controversial drug with a bad reputation. It is known on the streets as the date rape drug because of its use by sexual predators for illegal purposes.

In 2000 the U.S. government added GHB to a list of controlled substances that are illegal to manufacture or possess. But, because of its effectiveness in clinical trials (drug tests on human subjects), in 2002 a form of GHB called sodium oxybate was approved by the Food and Drug Administration for treating narcolepsy.

Due to safety concerns, patients can only get a limited amount of the drug. Sodium oxybate is potentially addictive, and withdrawal can be difficult, and it can cause a number of unpleasant side effects. It is, therefore, typically reserved for severe cases in which other medications have proven to be ineffective.

patients to find the most effective and comfortable mask for each individual. PAP therapy is 90 percent effective for patients who use it on a nightly basis. However, only 50 percent of sleep apnea patients stick with the treatment. Patients report having trouble adjusting to sleeping with the mask on, to the cool air blowing against their faces, and to the whooshing sound the blower makes. Despite these drawbacks, when patients commit to the therapy it can change their lives. As a sleep apnea sufferer named Bill explains: "It's been a little over a month since I started using a CPAP and I have been sleeping *much* better and will not sleep without my CPAP machine. It has enabled me to watch TV shows and not fall asleep. I also feel like I have more energy and walked to the store (a five to ten minute walk one way) whereas before I would have driven my truck. Since using the CPAP I feel like I have *much* more energy!"[27]

Other Therapies

Other sleep disorders require different treatments. Patients with bruxism are often fitted with a customized dental guard that is worn during sleep. Dental guards are similar to athletic mouth guards. They are usually made of plastic and fit over some or all of the patient's upper and/or lower teeth. Dental guards provide a cushion between the upper and lower teeth, reducing teeth grinding and protecting the teeth and jaw.

People with circadian rhythm disorders are often prescribed light therapy. It helps them reset their circadian clocks. Light therapy involves the use of a light box, a device that emits

A technician holds a plastic dental guard that is worn during sleep by people who grind their teeth in order to protect their jaw and teeth.

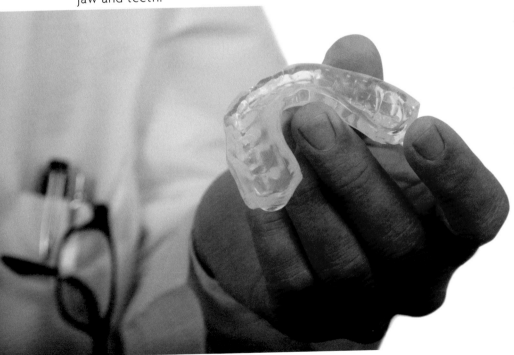

light that resembles sunlight. Light boxes look like small LED panels and come in many designs. Patients place the light box by their bed at a prescribed distance from their face and set it to turn on around 7 A.M. The bright light emitted by the box signals the brain to wake up. In addition, patients are advised to avoid bright light exposure in the evening. This routine gradually helps patients to fall asleep and awaken at more normal hours.

Sleep Disorder Medicines

A variety of medicines are also used to treat sleep disorders. The type of medication depends on the particular disorder and the patient's symptoms. For instance, stimulants, drugs that promote wakefulness and counteract daytime sleepiness, are often prescribed for people with narcolepsy. Modafinil is one of the newest and most popular medications in this category. Scientists are unclear about exactly how the drug works. It appears to act on the hypothalamus, the part of the brain that regulates sleepiness and wakefulness.

Patients take the drug first thing in the morning. Its effects wear off by the time they go to bed at night. Like all stimulants, modafinil can raise blood pressure, so it can be dangerous for patients with heart problems.

Patients who have cataplexy may be prescribed an antidepressant medication. Antidepressants are primarily prescribed to control depression, but they also suppress REM sleep and reduce cataplexy episodes.

Hypnotics

Low doses of certain antidepressants that produce sleepiness are also prescribed for patients with insomnia, as are drugs known as hypnotics. Hypnotics come in two forms: benzodiazepines and non-benzodiazepines, or Z-drugs. Benzodiazepines were developed much earlier than non-benzodiazepines, which were developed in the 1990s. Both classes of hypnotics work by attaching to receptors on brain cells involved in triggering sleepiness. But the two classes of hypnotics are chemically dif-

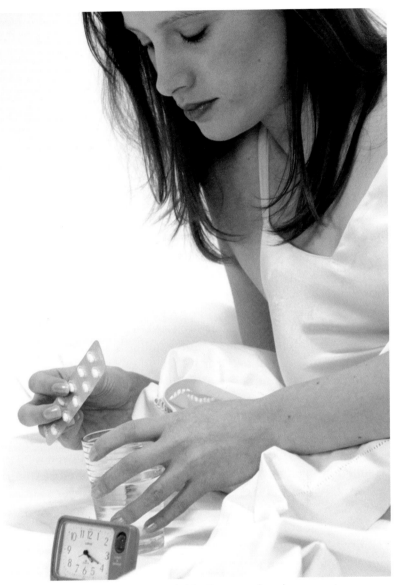

A range of medicines are available for people who experience sleep disorders.

ferent. Benzodiazepines, such as diazepam (Valium) and alprazolam (Xanax), do not leave the body as quickly as do Z-drugs. They provide sleepers with a full night's sleep, but, because benzodiazepines can remain in the bloodstream for forty-eight to seventy-two hours, they can cause daytime sleepiness and memory loss. Also, over time, patients build up a tolerance to benzodiazepines, which means they have to keep increasing their dosage for the medication to be effective. In addition, benzodiazepines are addictive, causing unpleasant withdrawal symptoms. And, even when withdrawal symptoms have disappeared, many people experience long-term rebound insomnia, a condition in which insomnia symptoms return more severely than ever.

Non-benzodiazepines are less damaging. They include zolpidem (Ambien), zaleplon (Sonata), and eszopiclone (Lunesta). These drugs help people fall asleep quickly. They leave the body within about four or five hours, which allows individuals with sleep maintenance insomnia to take a pill in the middle of the night. On the other hand, because they leave the body quickly, they have a short duration of effectiveness, meaning that users may awaken too early. As author Gayle Greene explains: "After the two to four hours of sleep I can usually get on my own, I nibble off three to five milligrams from [a Z-drug] pill. It gives me about an hour [of sleep] per milligram, up to a maximum of five hours—even if I take ten or fifteen milligrams I never get more than five hours."[28]

Other problems arise because of the odd effect Z-drugs have on some patients' behavior. Patients have reported bizarre parasomnia episodes like eating, cooking, driving, Internet shopping, telephoning, committing crimes, setting fires, and engaging in sexual activities while under the influence of Z-drugs. "I almost drove off a cliff 50 yards from my house,"[29] explains actor Jack Nicholson about his experience with a Z-drug.

Z-drugs are not meant to be taken every night. When individuals take them nightly for more than two weeks, they can build up a tolerance to the medication. And, although Z-drugs are not physically addictive, people can develop a psychological dependence on them. Despite these risks, Z-drugs help millions of people sleep. As Greene explains, "The difference between the two to four hours I get on my own and the seven to eight hours I can get with a few milligrams of Ambien is the difference between walking and hobbling through life."[30]

Treating Sleep Problems with Aromatherapy

Practitioners of the traditional medicine of India known as Ayurveda have used aromatherapy for centuries to treat sleep problems. In aromatherapy, patients inhale the aroma of oils distilled from plants having sleep-inducing properties. The oils are usually placed in a special diffuser where they heat up and disperse into the air as a mist. Patients inhale the mist into their bloodstreams through their lungs.

Different scents produce different effects. Lavender and jasmine are the most commonly used scents for treating sleeplessness. Both contain chemicals that appear to have a calming, mildly sedating effect on the body. In a 2002 study, researchers at Wheeling Jesuit University in West Virginia compared the effect the scent of jasmine, lavender, and no scent at all had on the sleep of subjects for three nights. The researchers found that the sleepers in the jasmine- and lavender-scented rooms slept better and were less anxious upon waking than the subjects in the unscented rooms. The sleepers in the jasmine-scented room also reported greater afternoon alertness the following day than any of the other subjects.

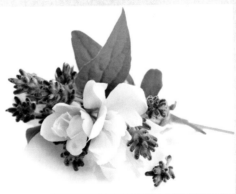

The scents of lavender and jasmine are commonly used to promote sleep.

Cognitive Behavioral Therapy

Cognitive behavioral therapy, or CBT, is another treatment for insomnia. It may be combined with medication or administered alone. In cognitive behavioral therapy, patients work with a psychologist to help correct thought patterns and behaviors that can cause or worsen insomnia. According to Dr. Nancy Foldvary-Schaefer, the director of the Cleveland Clinic Sleep Disorders Center, "The goal of CBT is to empower patients and help them gain control over sleep through education."[31]

In sessions with a psychologist, patients learn a variety of techniques that are used to correct their sleep patterns. Relaxation training is among these. Relaxation training includes practicing deep breathing at bedtime, which calms the body and lessens feelings of anxiety associated with not being able to sleep. Visualization is another relaxation practice. In visualization, individuals substitute pleasant images of themselves relaxing and falling asleep for stressful images that keep them awake.

Sleep restriction therapy is another technique. It improves patients' sleep efficiency; that is, the percentage of time spent in bed asleep. For example, if a person spends eight hours in bed but only sleeps for four hours, their sleep efficiency is 50 percent. People without sleep problems average 90 percent sleep efficiency.

Sleep restriction therapy involves matching the amount of time spent in bed with sleep time. So, if individuals spend eight hours in bed, but only five sleeping, sleep restriction therapy restricts their time in bed to five hours. Since patients with insomnia often underestimate the amount of time they spend sleeping, sleep restriction therapy causes them to feel sleepier than usual, raising their sleep drive. As a result, they fall asleep faster and sleep more deeply the next night. And, as they start sleeping better they begin to associate their bed with sleep instead of anxiety-inducing insomnia symptoms. As sleep efficiency increases, patients increase their time in bed by fifteen-minute increments with the goal of reaching 85 percent sleep efficiency. As sleep expert John Cline explains:

Sleep restriction, or perhaps more accurately, bed restriction, is based on the assumption that sleep deprivation will increase the drive to sleep and to remain asleep. This may not fit with the experience of those with insomnia for whom sleep seems impossible no matter how long they have not slept. It does make sense, however, when you consider that people with insomnia often underestimate the amount of sleep they are getting, in part because they misinterpret light sleep as wakefulness. Another effect that sleep restriction has is to break up the relationship between being in bed and being awake. Over time, being in bed while awake can lead to conditioning effects such that the bed becomes a conditioned stimulus for arousal. By limiting the amount of time in bed to approximately the amount of time spent sleeping, the bed becomes a conditioned stimulus for sleep. Just getting in bed can then elicit sleep rather than arousal.[32]

People with sleep disorders are often advised to refrain from reading, watching television, or using electronics while in bed so that their brains associate their beds only with relaxation and sleep.

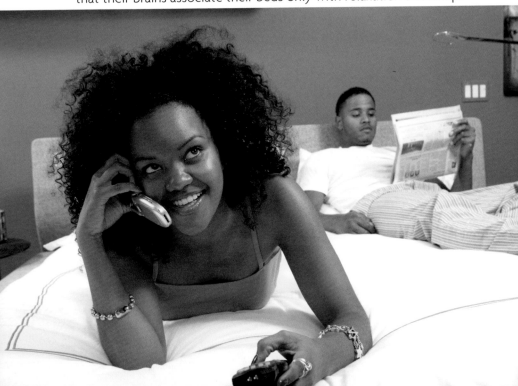

Stimulus control therapy also conditions patients to associate their beds with relaxation and sleep. In stimulus control therapy patients are trained to use their bed only for sleep or intimate relations. All other activities, including watching television, eating, reading, and texting, are done in another room. When patients go to bed, if they cannot fall asleep or if they wake up during the night and cannot fall back to sleep, they must move to another room until they feel sleepy. Proponents say that associating the bedroom only with sleep helps people fall asleep more rapidly and alleviates much of the stress linked to insomnia.

Nontraditional Treatments

Traditional treatments for sleep disorders are not effective for every patient. Even if these methods do help, some individuals are uncomfortable with the health risks that prescription sleep medications pose. Others find practices like stimulus control therapy too strict and demanding. Consequently, many people with sleep disorders turn to nontraditional, alternative treatments. Alternative treatments are treatments that are not widely accepted by the traditional medical community in the United States. Unlike conventional treatments, nontraditional medications are not subject to rigorous testing and careful regulation by the U.S. Food and Drug Administration (FDA). As a result, the purity or effectiveness of the medication or supplement may be suspect.

Despite this, many individuals find that alternative treatments such as melatonin supplements and herbal remedies help them to sleep. Melatonin supplements increase the levels of the hormone the brain secretes to promote sleep. The melatonin in the supplement is usually made synthetically. Melatonin supplements appear to help regulate sleep/waking patterns and are most effective in treating circadian rhythm disorders; however, the supplements have reportedly caused nightmares, headaches, daytime grogginess, depression, and mood swings in some users.

Herbal treatments are also popular. Herbs have been used to promote sleep for thousands of years. Teas made from chamo-

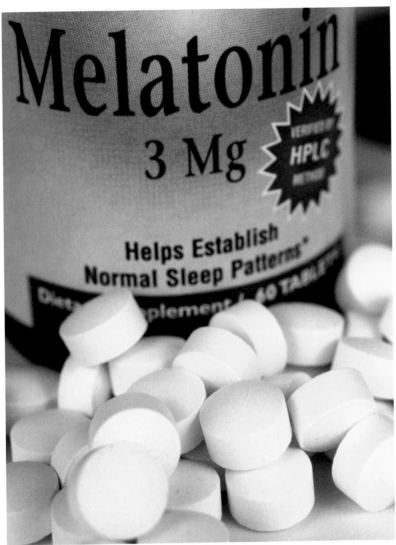

Melatonin supplements are among several alternative medicine treatments used to help people manage sleep disorders.

mile or valerian root, in particular, contain chemicals that produce a calming effect that promotes sleep. Herbs, however, are powerful substances. Valerian root and chamomile can cause allergic reactions and side effects like headaches, skin rash, and indigestion. Moreover, the chemicals in herbs can negatively interact with prescribed medications. So, it is best for patients to check with their doctors before using herbal remedies.

Over-the-counter sleep aids, which are less powerful than prescription medications or herbs, are another option. Americans spend millions of dollars each year on these products. Most contain antihistamines, chemicals that are used to treat allergies and nasal congestion and also cause sleepiness as a side effect. These products are most effective for occasional use only, but, like any medication, they can cause unpleasant side effects.

Clearly, no treatment, whether traditional or nontraditional, is effective for every patient. The health risks or discomfort some treatments present discourage many patients from using them. Despite these drawbacks, seeking diagnosis and experimenting with different treatments under the supervision of a health care professional is an important step in counteracting the debilitating effects of sleep disorders.

CHAPTER FOUR

Adopting Good Sleep Strategies

Getting enough good-quality sleep makes a tremendous difference in a person's health and well-being. People with sleep disorders improve their sleep by taking a number of steps. Among these steps are a variety of strategies that often involve lifestyle changes.

Sleep Hygiene

One of the most important steps to improving sleep is practicing good sleep hygiene. *Sleep hygiene* is a term that refers to healthful habits that promote sleep. One of these habits is keeping a consistent sleep schedule with a regular bedtime and awakening time. This applies to weekdays and weekends. Keeping a regular sleep schedule helps condition the brain to fall asleep at an appropriate time and helps the body's circadian clock to function properly. An article on the University of Maryland Medical Center's website advises: "Do not be one of those people who allows bedtime and awakening time to drift. The body 'gets used' to falling asleep at a certain time, but only if this is relatively fixed. Even if you are retired or not working, this is an essential component of good sleeping habits."[33]

Avoiding long naps during the day is another good sleep hygiene practice. If individuals sleep too much during the day, they are not tired at night. Experts advise people who cannot get through the day without napping to limit their nap times to no more than forty minutes and to nap before 3 P.M., so they will be tired at their regular bedtimes.

Restricting Stimulating Substances

Practicing good sleep hygiene also involves restricting consumption of stimulating substances like alcohol, tobacco, and caffeine. Many people think that drinking an alcoholic beverage before bedtime helps them sleep. Alcohol does have a sleep-inducing effect, which makes it easier for individuals to fall asleep initially; however, as alcohol is processed by the body it produces a stimulant, or wake-up, effect, which increases the time people spend awake during the night. Alcohol also disrupts normal sleep cycles and reduces rapid-eye-movement, or REM, sleep. A 2011 University of Michigan study helped confirm this. The study looked at the effect of alcohol on sleep. Researchers had ninety-three healthy subjects drink either an intoxicating amount of alcohol or a placebo—sugar water that looked and tasted like an alcoholic beverage—shortly before bedtime. Then, the subjects' sleep was monitored with a polysomnograph. The subjects who consumed alcohol had increased nighttime wakefulness, reduced total sleep time, reduced REM sleep, and felt less rested the next day compared with the subjects who consumed the placebo.

Making matters worse, because alcohol relaxes the upper airway, it can increase and worsen sleep apnea episodes. As sleep specialist Russell Rosenberg explains: "Millions of Americans suffer from obstructive sleep apnea, which can intensify after alcohol consumption. . . . Moderate to large amounts of alcohol consumed in the evening can lead to substantial narrowing of the airway, increasing the frequency and duration of breath holding episodes."[34]

Nicotine, a chemical found in tobacco, negatively affects sleep, too. It has a twofold effect on users. First it relaxes them; then it speeds up heartbeat, raises blood pressure, quickens breathing, and increases brain-wave activity. As a result, tobacco users wake up more frequently during the night than nonusers. During these arousals, some individuals get up and smoke, which makes matters worse. Smoking also harms the airway, making it more difficult for people with sleep apnea to breathe.

Caffeine is another stimulant. It blocks the release of sleep-inducing chemicals in the brain, reduces sleep duration, sleep efficiency, stage three, and REM sleep. At the same time, it raises blood pressure, heart rate, and brain activity.

Caffeine can be found in coffee, tea, soft drinks, and chocolate, as well as in some cold medicines and pain relievers. Caffeine stays in the body for a long time. Depending on the person, it can take from three to seven hours for one-half the caffeine in a cup of coffee to be eliminated from the body and

Tobacco and alcohol have a stimulant effect on the body, sometimes resulting in sleep problems for people who use them.

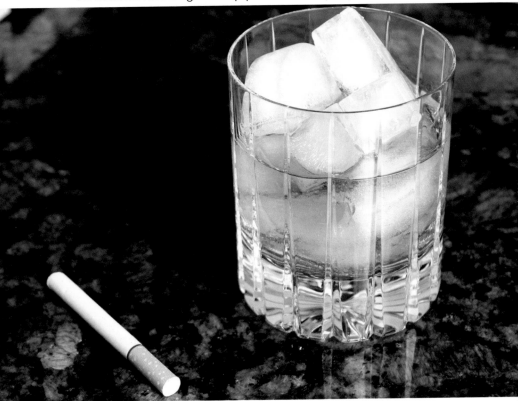

six to fourteen hours for all of it to be eliminated. According to author Gayle Greene: "If your last cup was at 1 P.M., you still have at 8 P.M. about half the drug left in your system, at 3 A.M. you have one-quarter of it, [and] at 10 A.M., one-eighth of it."[35] Consequently, when it comes to sleep, even one caffeinated beverage a day can cause problems, especially if it is consumed after twelve noon.

To complicate matters, because of the effect caffeine has on the body, the more caffeine an individual consumes the harder it is to eliminate. Therefore, according to nutritionist and blogger Julianne Taylor, "depending on how much caffeine you are consuming and your current medical status, the half-life of caffeine can increase to anything from 11–96 hours. Days!"[36] Not surprisingly, people who drink multiple caffeinated beverages per day often have insomnia. In some cases, their caffeine habit is the cause of their insomnia. In other cases, insomniacs use caffeine to energize themselves during the day, which worsens their insomnia symptoms at night. In both instances, eliminating caffeine consumption can drastically improve sleep patterns.

Food and Sleep

Just as people seeking a good night's sleep restrict their alcohol, tobacco, and caffeine intake before bedtime, they also are careful about the amount and types of food they eat before bedtime. As nutrition consultant Lisa Turner explains: "The foods we eat can dramatically affect how much, and how well, we sleep. Some calm and relax, some wake up the nervous system, and some just downright wire you for the night."[37]

Eating a heavy meal shortly before bedtime can negatively affect sleep. Usually the digestive system slows down during sleep. Eating a heavy meal at a late hour keeps the digestive system working long into the night. The results are often heartburn, gas, and nighttime visits to the bathroom, all of which cause discomfort and disrupt sleep. Also, "your body will be too busy digesting to focus on the restorative aspects of sleeping,"[38] explains nutritionist Beth Reardon. Sleep experts advise

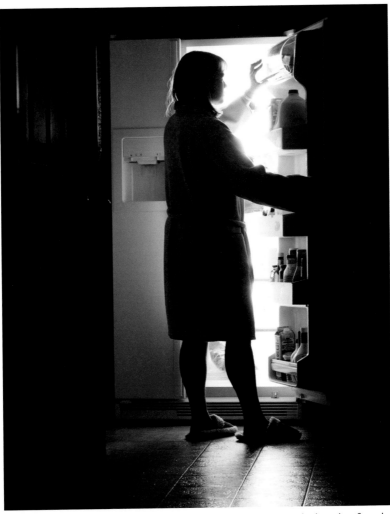

Sleep can be affected both negatively and positively by the food choices a person makes before bedtime. Foods that are hard to digest, high in fat and sugar, or spicy can disrupt sleep, while foods rich in tryptophan such as dairy products, turkey, and bananas can promote sleep.

individuals with sleep disorders to eat their last big meal at least four hours before bedtime.

Foods high in fat impact sleep in a similar manner. Fatty foods take longer to digest than other foods. A 2010 University of Pennsylvania study looked at the effect of fat intake on

Media Violence and Children's Sleep

According to a 2011 Seattle Children's Research Institute study, viewing violent movies, television programs, or video games can negatively affect children's sleep. With the help of parents, researchers monitored the media viewing habits and sleep of more than six hundred children aged three to five. The parents recorded the children's media viewing and sleep habits for a week, noting problems falling asleep, staying asleep, nightmares, trouble waking up in the morning, and tiredness during the day. The researchers found that the children who viewed violent media were more likely to have nightmares and other sleep problems, particularly if they viewed violent programs in the evening. Sleep problems increased with each additional hour of violent viewing. The researchers also found that the children who had a television in their bedroom watched an additional forty minutes of violent programming per day and were at the greatest risk of nightmares and sleep problems. Even slapstick violence in cartoons affected the young viewers' sleep. And, viewing violent programs with an adult or parent present did not change the results.

sleep duration in 459 women. The researchers found that the more fat the subjects ate, the less they slept.

Sugary foods are also troublesome. Sugar produces a rapid burst of energy followed by the release of stress hormones, which have a stimulating effect on the body. Spicy foods, too, have stimulating properties that disrupt sleep. Spicy foods can also cause indigestion and make body temperature rise, which interferes with sleep. "If you eat these foods late at night, they help promote acid reflux and can disturb sleep patterns because of that," explains Dr. Elizabeth Odstrcil of Baylor University Medical Center in Dallas. She adds, "Spicy foods are thought to raise body temperature and this causes more energy expenditure that's devoted to helping digest these foods instead of sleeping and your body resting."[39]

Other foods help promote sleep. These foods contain tryptophan, an amino acid (protein building block) that has a calming effect on the body. The body converts tryptophan into the hormones seratonin and melatonin, both of which induce sleep. Milk, cheese, yogurt, turkey, bananas, eggs, nuts, and seeds are all rich in tryptophan. Some people find that having a light snack containing tryptophan before bedtime helps them sleep better. To get the best results, they combine complex carbohydrates like whole-grain bread or cereal with tryptophan-rich foods. The combination increases tryptophan levels in the bloodstream and enhances its sleep-inducing properties. The addition of the mineral calcium, which is found in dairy products, helps the brain to efficiently use tryptophan to produce melatonin. Calcium is also a natural relaxant. This makes foods like milk, yogurt, and cheese that contain both calcium and tryptophan top sleep-inducing foods. People with sleep problems find that a bowl of cereal and milk; half of a turkey, cheese, or peanut butter sandwich with a glass of milk; a small bowl of yogurt with nuts; or whole-grain crackers and a glass of milk are all good sleep-inducing bedtime snacks.

Exercise and Sleep

Being physically active is another strategy that helps individuals sleep better. Exercise helps keep the body fit and healthy. It controls weight, which is especially helpful for people with sleep apnea, and reduces stress and anxiety. Exercise also tires the body, promoting a good night's sleep. A 2010 Northwestern University study looked at the effects of aerobic exercise—sustained physical activity such as running, walking, bicycling, dancing, and swimming—on a group of female insomniacs aged fifty-five and older. Half the subjects exercised for two twenty-minute sessions four times per week or one thirty- to forty-minute session four times per week. The other subjects acted as a control group. They did not exercise at all. Instead

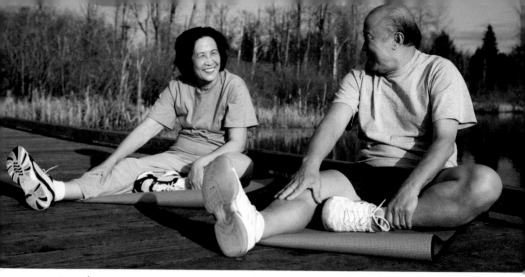

Regular exercise can promote healthy sleep patterns by keeping the body fit, reducing stress and anxiety, and making the body tired.

they participated in nonphysical activities such as playing cards. After sixteen weeks, the subjects who exercised showed a dramatic improvement in their sleep duration, sleep quality, and daytime energy levels, while the control group did not. The exercising group averaged an additional seventy-five minutes of sleep per night and a 33 percent reduction in nighttime arousals. The nonexercising group increased their amount of sleep time by twelve minutes a night and showed no difference in their amount of nighttime arousals.

Despite such benefits, since exercise increases heart and respiration rate and raises body temperature, problems can arise if individuals exercise too close to bedtime. For this reason, sleep experts say that to get the full benefit of exercise without the drawbacks, it is best to exercise at least four hours before bedtime. Dr. Michael Breus advises:

> For the most sleep-enhancing exercise routine, get moving in the morning, and get outside in the sunlight. This early-in-the-day exertion and exposure to sunlight will strengthen your circadian rhythms, helping you to feel more alert during the day—and sleepier at night. If morning exercise doesn't fit in your schedule, find another time during the day that does. To avoid exercise interfering with winding down for sleep at night, schedule your workout no closer than 4 hours before bedtime.[40]

Winding Down

Just as avoiding certain foods, drinks, and vigorous exercise right before bedtime helps improve sleep, so too does establishing a consistent, soothing pre-bedtime routine thirty minutes to one hour before bedtime. Such a routine helps relax the body and cues the brain that it is time for sleep. For example, if individuals take a warm bath and massage body lotion onto their skin every night before going to bed, their brains come to connect this routine with sleep and starts to wind down and prepare for sleep. As Harvard University's Lawrence Epstein explains: "Our body craves routine and likes to know what's coming."[41]

Any activity that relaxes the body and mind can be part of this pre-bedtime routine. Soothing activities such as listening to soft music, hair brushing, reading a book, taking a warm bath, or writing in a journal are all activities that help people relax and prepare for sleep. Some individuals keep a "worry" journal as part of their pre-bedtime routine. In it they record

Some sleep experts recommend that patients write in a journal as part of a pre-bedtime routine to help them manage stress and worries that may otherwise keep them awake.

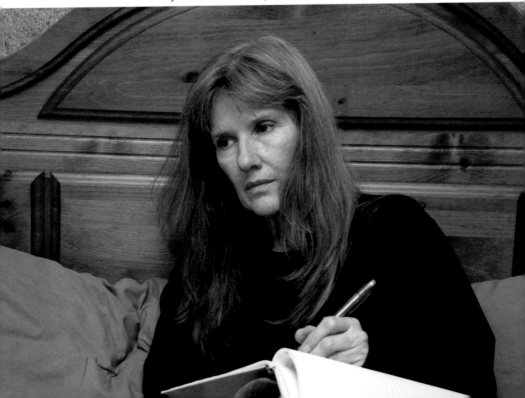

their daily worries. This practice helps individuals to keep worrisome thoughts from their minds once they close their eyes. If individuals find themselves worrying once they get into bed, they can tell themselves: "'I've dealt with that,' or 'I'm dealing with it.' This usually helps to create a "sense of relief,"[42] explains author and sleep specialist Stephanie Silberman.

Regulating the Body's Clock

Being aware of the body's reaction to light also helps people with sleep disorders sleep better. Exposure to light affects the body's natural circadian rhythm. Exposure to bright light at bedtime suppresses the production of melatonin, making it difficult to get to sleep, while limited exposure to light has the reverse effect. Brightly backlit devices, such as computers, tablets, and smartphones, are especially stimulating to the brain. Television watching, too, can have this effect. Using these devices before bedtime can disrupt an individual's circadian rhythm and delay sleep. Therefore, restricting their use close to bedtime is a strategy people use to improve sleep. As Breus explains:

> We're wired all the time, to our cell phones, computers, tablets, and televisions. These devices inevitably seem to find their way into our bedrooms, where they easily interfere with a good night's sleep. . . . Electronics in the bedroom disrupt sleep in a few ways. They emit light that can interfere with the body's circadian rhythm, and its production of the sleep-inducing hormone melatonin. Whether it's a late-night email, or a flurry of text messages, these devices provide mental stimulation—and stress—that can hinder sleep. To dramatically boost your relaxation levels at home, try turning off your electronics."[43]

Digital clocks with a blue light display can also disrupt people's circadian rhythm. Blue light is a bright form of light. It is very stimulating to the brain. Clocks with a red light display are less disruptive. But the presence of any clock near the bed can cause problems for people with sleep disorders, who often find

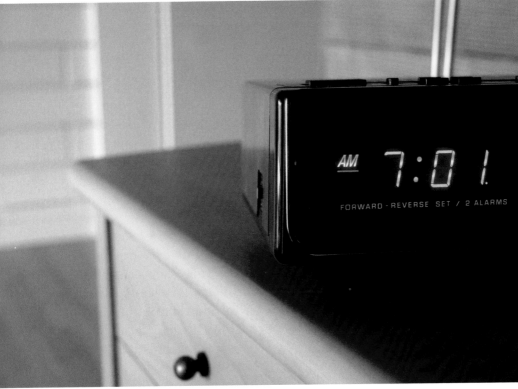

Digital clocks with a blue light display have been found to stimulate the brain and disrupt a person's circadian rhythm, thus making sleep more difficult.

themselves checking the clock throughout the night instead of trying to relax. Therefore, many people with sleep disorders remove all bedroom clocks from view.

Other strategies involving light, such as keeping the bedroom dark, also help. Sleeping with the lights on can signal the brain that it is time to be awake. Even little bits of light can pass through the eyelids to the brain, reducing or stopping the production of melatonin. Sleep experts say it is best to turn off all the lights and draw the blinds and curtains. Special blackout curtains are used by people like night-shift workers, whose work schedules require them to sleep during the day, or by individuals whose bedrooms face brightly lit streets. Blackout curtains look like regular curtains, but they contain an insulating panel that blocks out almost all light (hotel rooms usually have them). Alternatively, some sleepers wear an eye mask designed to help block out light.

Creating a Relaxing Sleep Environment

Besides keeping the bedroom dark, taking other steps to turn the bedroom into a relaxing place helps promote sleep. Keeping the bedroom temperature cool, between 65° and 70° F (18°–21°C), is most conducive to sleep. Temperatures too far below or above this range can cause restlessness. Indeed, respondents to a 2012 survey by the National Sleep Foundation rated a cool bedroom temperature as the most important bedroom factor contributing to a good night's sleep. Scientists are unclear why room temperature is so important. They know that people's body temperatures drop while they sleep. It is possible that having a cool room mimics this natural body temperature drop, making it easier for individuals to fall and stay asleep. This may also be why taking a warm bath about an hour before bedtime appears to encourage sleep. In addition to being soothing and relaxing, warm water raises the bather's body temperature, which drops when the bather gets out of the bath. This drop in temperature signals the body that it is time for sleep.

The bedroom's air quality is also vital to good sleep, especially for individuals with allergies. Dust, mold, pet hair, and other allergens on the bed linens or in the bedroom can make it hard for some people to breathe. Instead of resting, these individuals are likely to spend the night sneezing and coughing. Using an air purifier with a HEPA (high-efficiency particulate air) filter helps. It removes allergens from the air. And, since allergens tend to gather on soft surfaces, individuals find that removing stuffed toys and decorative pillows from the bed helps, as does keeping pets off the bed.

Sleeping with pets can interfere with sleep in other ways. If pets move around or snore, they may awaken sleepers. Other noises can be a problem, too. To help eliminate disrupting noises, many sleepers use a white-noise machine. It is a device that produces a soothing background sound that masks other, more disturbing sounds. A fan or an air conditioner also helps mask sound. Some people use earplugs to block out sound.

A warm bath before bedtime can encourage sleep because of its effects on body temperature.

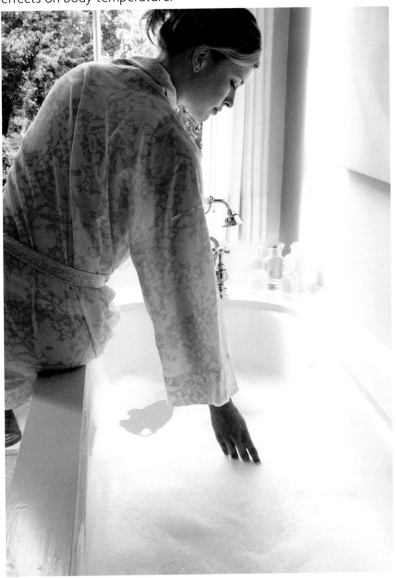

Rocking to Sleep

Parents often rock babies to sleep. A rocking motion may also help adults to fall asleep more easily. Researchers at the University of Switzerland in Geneva investigated the effect of rocking motion on the sleep of healthy adult male subjects, none of whom suffered from a sleep disorder. The subjects took two naps in specially designed beds that rocked like a hammock. During one nap the bed rocked. During the other the bed was still. The subjects' brain activity was monitored with an electro-encephalograph, or EEG, while they napped.

The researchers found that all the subjects fell asleep faster in the rocking beds, went from stage one to stage two sleep more quickly, and produced more slow-wave, deep-sleep brain waves associated with more restful, less fragmented sleep than while stationary. When questioned about the experience, the subjects said that sleeping in the rocking bed was more pleasant and re-laxing than sleeping in the stationary bed.

Based on these results, the researchers say that rocking motion helps individuals fall asleep more quickly and get a better quality of sleep. Individuals can get a similar effect by sleeping in a hammock.

The Bed

A clean, comfortable, welcoming bed is another important element in creating a soothing sleep environment. In fact, 71 percent of the respondents to the National Sleep Foundation survey said they sleep better on clean sheets, and 29 percent reported they go to sleep faster when they have clean sheets. Many people with sleep disorders find that frequently changing the sheets improves their sleep.

A comfortable, good-quality mattress and supportive pillows also promote sleep. A smooth, firm mattress provides the best support for a sleeper's back and neck. A sagging or lumpy mattress, on the other hand, can lead to nighttime arousals due to discomfort and cause individuals to wake up in the morning feeling stiff and sore. Many sleep experts suggest replacing mattresses every seven to ten years.

They also advise sleepers to replace their pillows often. Pillows support a sleeper's neck and head so that these body parts do not feel overstretched or squeezed. The right pillow can make a significant difference in how well a person sleeps. For example, Hector, a middle-aged man with sleep problems, found that a new pillow specially designed for people with sleep troubles improved his sleep quality: "I got a special pillow.

A bed with a supportive mattress, clean sheets, and comfortable pillows is conducive to sound sleep.

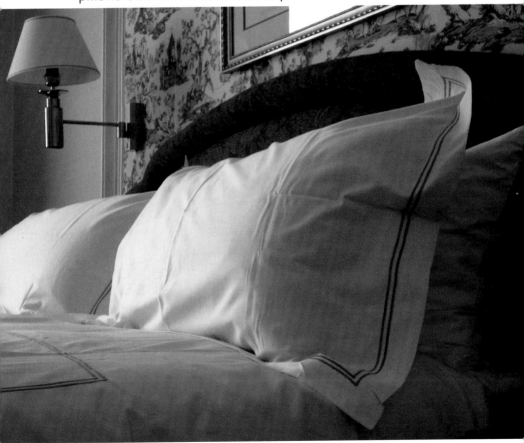

It is wonderful. I have an old neck and shoulder injury and this pillow supports my head and shoulders, so I am not in pain. I love it. I no longer wake up during the night. I am sleeping a lot better."[44]

From replacing pillows to practicing good sleep hygiene, people with sleep disorders may have to make many lifestyle changes to improve their sleep. But by doing so, they take control of their lives and improve their physical, mental, and emotional health.

CHAPTER FIVE

Looking to the Future

Sleep research is a relatively new field of study. Since so much about sleep is unknown, there are many areas to be studied. Some of the most interesting studies are focused on the mechanisms that underlie sleep and sleep disorders and on how sleep affects the body and the brain. Other studies examine the effect of diet on sleep disorders. Learning more about sleep should help scientists gain a better understanding of sleep disorders. This knowledge should lead to the development of new, more effective treatments.

Sleep Disorders and Genes

In a number of laboratory studies, scientists are trying to identify specific genes that regulate sleep. Many of these studies involve fruit flies. Because they are easier to study than more complex animals, fruit flies have been used in studies of genetics for many years. In fact, the fruit fly's genome, or complete genetic makeup, was fully mapped in 2000. So far, almost seventeen hundred genes associated with sleep in fruit flies have been identified. Researchers believe humans carry equivalent genes.

In 2012 researchers at Rockefeller University in New York City studied the sleep habits of twenty-one thousand fruit flies. The researchers noted that normally fruit flies sleep about 927 minutes—fifteen and three-quarter hours—a day. Some of the flies in the study, however, exhibited sleep habits much like those of humans with insomnia. These flies had problems staying asleep and slept only 317 minutes (about five and a half hours) a day. To find out whether a genetic mutation could be involved, the researchers studied the flies' genes. They found that all the sleep-deprived flies carried a mutant gene, which the researchers named "insomniac." The gene appears to be involved in homeostasis, the mechanism that signals the body to sleep when it is tired. The researchers are unclear exactly how the gene works. They think it is involved in breaking down proteins linked to sleep.

The researchers also investigated whether there was a link between reduced sleep and the fruit flies' lifespan. They found that the flies with the mutant insomniac gene lived only about two-thirds as long as the other flies.

The discovery of the insomniac gene is important because it is possible that human insomniacs carry an equivalent gene mutation. If this proves to be true, scientists could work on developing a method of modifying or replacing the mutant gene, or they could develop a drug that regulates the gene's actions. As researcher Nicholas Stavropoulos explains: "Sleep is a fundamental behavior in all animals, and it is poorly understood from a scientific standpoint. This work gives us several new clues about how sleep is controlled at the molecular level, and could prove useful in understanding and treating sleep disorders."[45]

In 2012 researchers at Emory University focused their attention on a different gene. The gene, which is known as BTBD9, had previously been linked to restless legs syndrome. The researchers examined the sleep behavior of fruit flies by putting individual flies in tubes with infrared sensors capable of detecting when a fly moved across the tube. The researchers considered the flies asleep if the insects did not move across the tubes for five minutes. They found that the fruit flies that carried mutations of the BTBD9 gene woke up more often and moved around more than the other flies.

Investigating further, the scientists found that the BTBD9 helps control the production of a protein involved in the storage of iron. Iron deficiencies have been linked to restless legs syndrome, which is likely a result of the mutant gene. Muta-

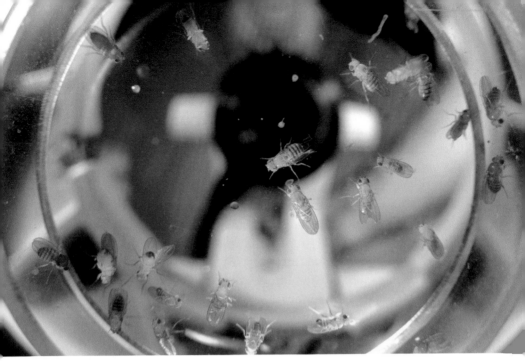

Laboratory studies with fruit flies have provided insight into a possible genetic basis for some sleep disorders.

tions in the gene also reduced levels of the brain chemical dopamine. Among its many functions, dopamine helps the brain control movement. Interestingly, a drug that, among other things, regulates dopamine production has recently been approved to treat restless legs syndrome.

Next, the researchers plan to investigate whether the gene has other functions that might be connected to the development of restless legs syndrome. Since the similarities between the effects of the mutant gene on the flies and in humans is striking, the scientists hope that their work will lead to a better understanding of restless legs syndrome, and more effective treatments. As researchers Subhabrata Sanyal and David Rye explain: "Flies and humans are distant from each other on the evolutionary tree, yet the same gene seems to be regulating a fundamental process in both organisms and affecting how soundly they sleep. . . . That's what's so remarkable about this result. The genetic context may be different, but the effects of the mutation are consistent with [restless legs syndrome] and the same modifying factors, such as dopamine and iron, are involved."[46]

Sleep and the Brain

Other researchers are taking a different approach. People with sleep disorders complain of mental fuzziness, memory problems, and difficulty learning. With this in mind, researchers are investigating the effect of sleep on the brain. One group of studies is focusing on the link between sleep, the formation and retention of memories, and learning.

Scientists believe that during stage three and rapid-eye-movement, or REM, sleep the brain replays experiences from the day, which strengthens memory. The brain gathers information throughout the day, which is stored in a network of nerve cells that connect communication pathways in the brain. There is, however, only so much physical space in the skull for the network. Many scientists theorize that in order to create space for new learning, during sleep the brain trims this neural network, discarding weaker connections and converting stronger connections into long-term memories. Two studies in 2009, conducted at Washington University in St. Louis and the University of Wisconsin at Madison, helped confirm this theory. In both studies, scientists examined the brains of fruit flies before and after sleep. Both studies found that after sleep the volume of connections between nerve cells in the brain decreased in size and number. "If this didn't happen, theoretically, over time, the brain would reach capacity and be unable to learn or remember new things," explains Washington University researcher Paul Shaw. "After a night's sleep, the next morning the brain wakes up and is ready to go, ready to acquire new information."[47]

Another Washington University study in 2011 established a link between sleep and the formation of long-term memories. In this study, the researchers altered a cluster of cells in the brains of fruit flies, which allowed the researchers to control the flies' sleep habits. To test whether sleep is connected to the formation of long-term memories, the researchers exposed male fruit flies to other male fruit flies that were altered to smell like female fruit flies. After a few unsuccessful attempts to mate, the unaltered male flies learned to ignore the altered flies. Then the researchers allowed some of the flies to sleep, while keeping others awake. The next day, the flies that slept did not attempt to mate with the altered flies. But the flies that were deprived of sleep did. The researchers concluded that the brain transforms new information into long-term memories during sleep and that without sleep, the brain is unable to convert short-term knowledge into long-term memories.

A 2011 Stanford University study found that the continuity of sleep was just as important in forming memories as the length of sleep. In this study, mice were exposed to new toys during the day. Then, the mice went to sleep. Half of the mice were allowed to sleep normally while the others were repeatedly

Learning While Dreaming

Sleep researchers are unsure why people dream. A 2010 study at Beth Israel Deaconess Medical Center in Boston suggests that dreaming helps learning. In this study, ninety-nine adult subjects spent an hour trying to get through a virtual maze. Half the subjects then slept for ninety minutes, and half relaxed while awake. During the ninety minutes, the subjects were awakened or interrupted and asked to describe their dreams or thoughts. When the rest period was up, all the subjects tried to solve the maze again. The subjects who had stayed awake showed no improvement in their ability to solve the maze. The subjects who had slept but did not report any maze-related dreams improved slightly. The subjects who reported dreaming about the maze showed a significant improvement. The difference in their scores on the maze before and after dreaming was ten times higher. Interestingly, the dreamers did not dream about solving the maze, but the maze was simply part of their dream. For example, one subject dreamt about the music played during the task, while another dreamt about meeting people in the maze. The researchers theorize that dreams may be the brain's way of improving learning and creatively solving problems.

awakened. Both groups slept for the same amount of time. The next day, the mice were exposed to brand-new toys. The mice that slept continuously explored the new toys while ignoring the toys from the day before, while the mice whose sleep was disrupted explored the old toys as if they were unfamiliar.

While these studies help explain problems with memory and learning connected with sleep disorders, a 2011 Washington University study may have found a treatment that can lessen these problems. In this study, researchers once again looked at the link between sleep deprivation, memory formation, and learning in fruit flies. The scientists paired a negative stimulus, quinine, which the flies dislike, with a positive stimulus, light, which attracts the flies. Then they gave the flies a choice of entering a dark tube without quinine or a lighted tube with quinine. The flies that slept normally learned to avoid the lighted tube, while the sleep-deprived flies did not.

While studying the flies, the researchers found that sleep deprivation caused the suppression of a protein known as NOTCH in the fruit flies' brains. The researchers found a similar decrease in NOTCH in sleep-deprived humans. Curious about what role NOTCH might play in learning, the researchers artificially increased the production of NOTCH in the sleep-deprived flies and tested their ability to learn. The flies were now able to learn just as quickly as the flies that slept normally. According to Shaw, "To our surprise, we found if NOTCH activity is boosted in the brains of sleep-deprived fruit flies, the flies can continue to stay sharp and learn after sleep deprivation. They behave as if they had a full night's sleep."[48]

Based on this study, the scientists are hoping to develop treatments that target either the gene that suppresses NOTCH or the part of the brain where NOTCH is produced. Such treatment would help reduce memory and learning problems caused by sleep disorders.

Sleep Apnea and Dementia

Reduced cognitive abilities and impairment of memory are also connected to dementia, a disorder that affects the brain. Because lack of good-quality sleep affects the formation of

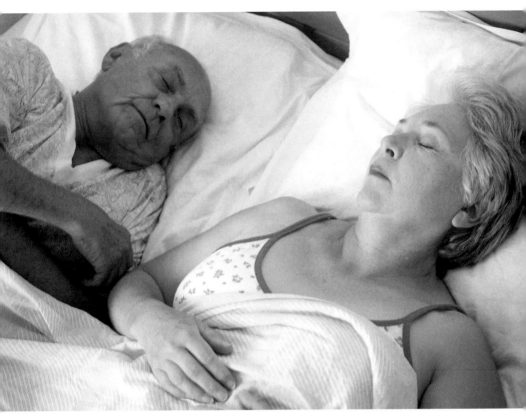

Researchers have discovered a correlation between sleep apnea and dementia in otherwise healthy older adults.

memories, and lack of oxygen is harmful to the brain, scientists at the University of California at San Francisco investigated whether there was a link between the development of dementia and sleep apnea. The study began in 2006, when the researchers monitored the sleep of 298 physically and mentally healthy women with an average age of eighty-two. Sleep monitoring showed that 105 of the subjects had sleep apnea. The women were also administered tests that measured their memory and cognitive abilities. All the subjects were reexamined five years later. None of the subjects with sleep apnea had received treatment for the condition in the interim. After controlling for variables such as the presence of other diseases, the use of certain medicines, and body weight that might impact the results, the researchers found that the subjects with sleep apnea were 85 percent more likely to have developed dementia or mild cognitive impairment than the other subjects.

Since the study monitored the subjects for only one night, the results are not conclusive. But they do show a correlation between sleep apnea and dementia. Says study leader Kristine Yaffe:

> This is the first study to show that sleep apnea may lead to cognitive impairment. It suggests that there is a biological connection between sleep and cognition and also suggests that treatment of sleep apnea might help prevent or delay the onset of dementia in older adults. While we cannot conclude from these results that [sleep-disordered breathing] causes cognitive impairment, our study suggests that it may at least be a contributing factor.[49]

If further studies substantiate the connection, it is likely that in the future people with sleep apnea will be monitored for dementia symptoms. And, because the link between sleep apnea and dementia shows how vital it is that people with sleep apnea get and stick with treatment, it should also lead to the development of newer sleep apnea treatments that more patients can tolerate.

Sleep and Emotions

Other researchers are investigating whether sleep disorders impact emotions. Individuals with sleep disorders often complain that lack of good-quality sleep causes them to feel cranky, agitated, and overemotional. A 2011 University of California at Berkeley study looked at the connection between sleep problems and emotions. The results of the study suggest that emotional experiences are processed during REM sleep, so that unpleasant experiences feel less painful and emotionally charged upon waking.

In this study, researchers divided thirty-five adult subjects into two groups. Both groups were shown a series of pictures designed to produce powerful negative emotions. As they viewed the pictures, the subjects' brain activity was monitored

Careers in Sleep Science

Individuals trained in sleep science are currently in high demand in the job market and should continue to be in the future. Individuals interested in sleep can train to be physicians with a specialty in sleep disorders. This requires a four-year college degree followed by eight years of medical training. Training as a psychologist is another path to a career in sleep science. Psychologists must have a minimum of a four-year college degree. Scientists who specialize in sleep research also need a minimum of a four-year college degree. However, most scientists and psychologists go on to get advanced degrees.

There are not many jobs for nurses specifically devoted to sleep disorders. But nurses interested in sleep can work for medical practices in related medical fields, including psychiatry, pulmonology (diseases of the respiratory system, including sleep apnea), and general medical practices. Nurses need either a two-year or a four-year degree in nursing.

Sleep lab technicians or polysomnography technologists also need a two-year associate's degree from an accredited training program. Many community colleges offer certification in polysomnography. Sleep lab technologists can earn between forty thousand dollars and eighty thousand dollars a year.

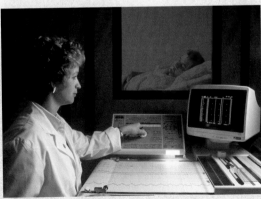

Sleep lab technicians attend an accredited training program and may hold an associate's degree.

with functional magnetic resonance imaging, or fMRI. Both groups viewed the pictures twice with a twelve-hour break between viewing. One group viewed the pictures in the morning and again in the evening, without sleeping in between. The other group viewed the pictures in the evening, then slept a full night during which their sleep was monitored before viewing the pictures again in the morning. The subjects who slept reported a decreased emotional reaction upon viewing the pictures the second time and their MRIs showed a significant decrease in activity in the region of the brain involved in emotions. The subjects who did not sleep between viewings had no change in emotional reaction. The researchers noted that during REM sleep, the sleepers' brains suppressed the release of a chemical associated with stress and arousal as if a function of REM sleep was to soothe the brain of stressful experiences.

Continued studies into the relationship of REM sleep and emotions are likely. "A greater understanding of this possible connection," explains Dr. Michael Breus, "could have a profound effect on how we view, and treat, sleep problems and the secondary effects of sleeplessness."[50]

Sleep Disorders and Emotional Problems in Children

Another group of scientists are investigating whether there is a connection between sleep disorders and emotional and behavioral problems in children. A study at Albert Einstein College of Medicine in New York City followed eleven thousand children for six years, ending in 2012. At various intervals, the subjects' parents answered a questionnaire about the children's sleep habits and another about the children's behavior. The latter assessed hyperactivity, inattentiveness, emotional issues, aggressiveness, and social skills. The researchers found the children with sleep-disordered breathing were at significantly greater risk of being hyperactive and having other emotional problems. As researcher Karen Bonuck explains:

> We found that children with sleep-disordered breathing were from 40 to 100 percent more likely to develop neu-

robehavioral problems by age 7, compared with children without breathing problems. . . . This is the strongest evidence to date that snoring, mouth breathing, and apnea can have serious behavioral and social-emotional consequences for children. Parents and pediatricians alike should be paying closer attention to sleep-disordered breathing in young children, perhaps as early as the first year of life.[51]

A 2011 University of Michigan study yielded similar results. In this study, researchers compiled information on 341 elementary-school-aged children's sleep and behavioral habits. The researchers found that the subjects who had sleep problems, particularly

Mouth breathing, snoring, and sleep apnea among children have been tied to emotional and behavioral problems, including aggressiveness and poor impulse control.

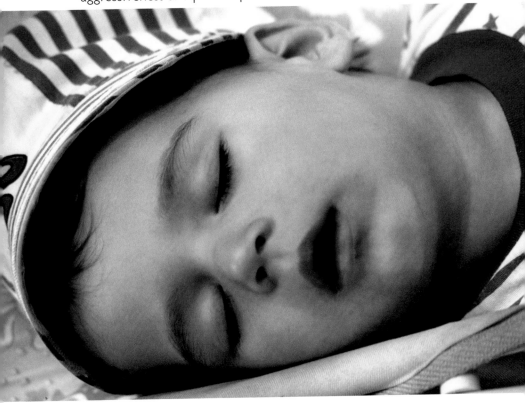

sleep-disordered breathing, were twice as likely to have behavioral problems like disruptive behavior, aggressiveness, and poor impulse control.

Neither study proves that sleep disorders cause emotional and behavioral problems in children, but they do suggest a strong link. Michigan researcher Dr. Louise O'Brien explains: "We can't look at cause and effect, but it certainly fits with the data that's out in the literature already. The hypothesis is that impaired sleep does affect areas of the brain. If that's disrupted, then emotional regulation and decision-making capabilities are impaired. The fact that sleepiness was so predictive of behavioral issues has implications for all children."[52]

Light Sleepers Versus Heavy Sleepers

Still focusing on the relationship between sleep and the brain, in 2010 researchers at Harvard Medical School investigated the part the brain plays in making people light or heavy sleepers. Light sleepers, many of whom suffer from insomnia, are easily awakened by external stimuli. Heavy sleepers are less likely to be disturbed.

In this study, researchers monitored the brain waves of twelve healthy adult subjects while they slept for three nights, focusing their attention on the number of sleep spindles, or pulses, that the sleepers' thalamuses produced. The thalamus is a part of the brain involved in processing external stimuli. The first night, the subjects' sleep was undisturbed by external stimuli. On the next two nights, the subjects were exposed to different sounds at progressively louder volumes, including the sound of car traffic, an airplane taking off, doors slamming, and toilets flushing. The researchers noted that the subjects whose thalamus produced the most sleep spindles were more likely to sleep through the sounds than sleepers who produced fewer spindles. They concluded that more spindles protected individuals from sleep disturbances.

The researchers plan more studies. Confirmation of their findings should lead to the development of drugs that can increase the number of spindles and give lighter sleepers a better

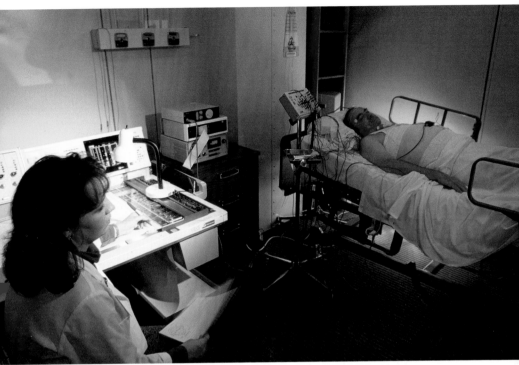

A technician observes a patient during a sleep study. Research provides information scientists can use to better understand and treat sleep disorders and other health impacts of sleep.

night's rest. According to researcher Dr. Jeffrey Ellenbogen, "The name of the game in sleep is stacking the cards in your favor, and one of those cards is having a quiet environment. When it's not quiet, we need to figure out how to block that sound from getting the brain to cause you to wake up. And hopefully brain-based solutions will one day be an option for protecting sleepers from losing sleep every night."[53]

Diet and Sleep Disorders

Other scientists are taking a completely different approach. They are investigating whether what individuals eat can relieve sleep disorders. In this regard, a 2011 study at the University of Crete in Greece is particularly interesting. In this study, researchers theorized that eating a Mediterranean-style diet

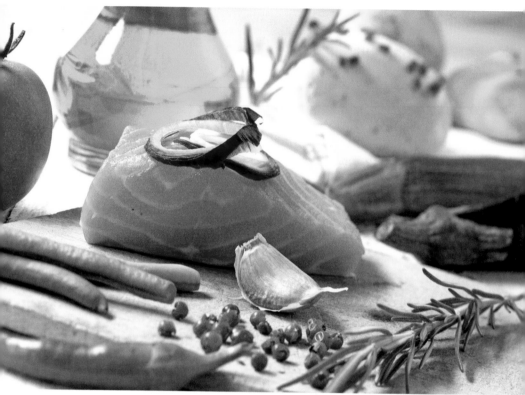

A Mediterranean diet, which is rich in fish, healthy oils, vegetables, fruits, whole grains, and nuts, is associated with reducing sleep apnea.

could reduce sleep apnea episodes. A Mediterranean diet is rich in fruit, vegetables, fish, whole grains, nuts and seeds, and healthy fats such as olive oil. It is considered to be very healthful and appears to help protect the body from a number of diseases.

To test their theory, the researchers divided forty obese patients with sleep apnea into two groups. One group followed a low-calorie diet for six months. The other followed a Mediterranean diet. Both groups were encouraged to exercise for thirty minutes a day, and all the subjects were administered continuous positive airway pressure, or CPAP, treatment. The subjects' sleep was monitored at the start of the study and again six months later. The researchers found that the subjects that followed the Mediterranean diet had a reduced number of apnea episodes, while the other group did not.

Further studies are planned. Depending on the results, it is quite possible that someday this type of diet may be part of sleep apnea treatment. In the meantime, since a Mediterranean diet is quite healthful in itself, people with sleep apnea can consider adopting the diet in an effort to ease their symptoms.

It is clear that the field of sleep research is booming. With each passing day, the many mysteries surrounding sleep are being revealed. All that is being learned should lead to a better understanding of sleep disorders and, as a result, better sleep for millions of sleep-deprived people.

Notes

Introduction: A Growing Problem

1. Geraint Vincent. "Bad Tempered, Forgetful, and Too Scared to Call a Friend: My Life as an Insomniac." *Observer* (London), November 12, 2011. www.guardian.co .uk/lifeandstyle/2011/nov/13/insomnia-sleep-deprivation -geraint-vincent.
2. Gretchen Rubin. "Get More Sleep and Improve Your Mood." *Good Housekeeping*, no date. www.goodhouse keeping.com/health/wellness/happiness-project-sleep -well.
3. Quoted in Anita Bruzzese. "Going Nonstop All Day Can Thwart Productivity on the Job." *USA Today*, July 7, 2010. www.usatoday.com/money/jobcenter/workplace /bruzzese/2010-07-07-take-time-to-rest_N.htm.
4. D.T. Max. "The Secrets of Sleep." *National Geographic*, May 2010, p. 74.

Chapter One: A Basic Need

5. Quoted in Jann Gumbiner. "Why Sleep Is Important." *Psychology Today*, February 28, 2012. www.psychology today.com/blog/the-teenage-mind/201202/why-sleep-is -important.
6. Nancy Foldvary-Schaefer. *The Cleveland Clinic Guide to Sleep Disorders*. New York: Kaplan, 2009, p. 6.
7. Quoted in Shaun Dreisbach. "Are You Living in Sleep Debt?" *Glamour*, August 2011, p. 99.
8. Quoted in Alice Park. "Lack of Sleep Linked to Heart Problems." *Time*, December 23, 2008. www.time.com/time /health/article/0,8599,1868406,00.html.
9. Quoted in Gayle Greene. *Insomniac*. Berkeley: University of California Press, 2008, p. 108.
10. Greene. *Insomniac*, pp. 109–110.

Chapter Two: Many Disorders

11. Quoted in Greene. *Insomniac*, p. 122.

12. Quoted in Greene. *Insomniac*, p. 9.

13. Quoted in Neurology and Sleep Medicine Consultants of Houston and the Houston Sleep Center. "Share Your Sleep Story." www.houstonsleepcenter.com/projectsleep .html.

14. Quoted in Stephen Galloway. "George Clooney: The Private Life of a Superstar." *Hollywood Reporter*, February 24, 2012, p. 44. www.hollywoodreporter.com/news/george -clooney-oscars-brad-pitt-stacy-keibler-descendants-290691.

15. Talk About Sleep. "Patient Stories—Mike's Story." www .talkaboutsleep.com/third_tier/patient_stories_sleepapnea _mike.htm.

16. Talk About Sleep. "Patient Stories—Mike's Story."

17. Quoted in Esther Crain. "Tingly Jumpy Legs When You Lie Down." *Cosmopolitan*, January 2012, p. 111.

18. Laura Linley. "Sleepy Kids: Understanding Pediatric Sleep Disorders." *Focus: Journal for Respiratory Care & Sleep Medicine*, Fall 2011, p. 17.

19. An EP User. "I Sleep Walk." Experience Project, February 12, 2012. www.experienceproject.com/stories/Sleep-Walk /2059863.

20. Quoted in Neurology and Sleep Medicine Consultants of Houston and the Houston Sleep Center. "Share Your Sleep Story."

21. John Cline. "Delayed Sleep Phase Syndrome." *Psychology Today*, August 30, 2009. www.psychologytoday.com/blog /sleepless-in-america/200908/delayed-sleep-phase.

22. Stephanie Handy and Tracy R. Nasca. "Life with Narcolepsy." Talk About Sleep, October 12, 2010. www.talk aboutsleep.com/sleep-disorders/2010/10/Life-With-Narco lepsy.htm.

23. Quoted in Ariel Neuman. "GHB's Path to Legitimacy: An Administrative and Legislative History of Xyrem." LEDA at Harvard Law School, April 2004. http://leda.law.harvard .edu/leda/data/629/Neuman.html.

24. Handy and Nasca. "Life with Narcolepsy."

Chapter Three: Diagnosis and Treatment

25. Eric Fields. "My Night in the Lab: What a Sleep Study Really Feels Like." *Health*, July 30, 2008. www.health.com /health/condition-article/0,,20215341,00.html.
26. Talk About Sleep. "Patient Stories—Tracy's Story." www .talkaboutsleep.com/third_tier/patient_stories_sleepapnea _tracy.htm.
27. Talk About Sleep. "Patient Stories—Bill's Story." www.talk aboutsleep.com/third_tier/patient_stories_sleepapnea_bill .htm.
28. Greene. *Insomniac*, p. 191.
29. Quoted in Tom Pettifor. "Jack Nicholson: I Warned Heath Ledger." *Mirror* (London), January 24, 2008. www.mirror .co.uk/news/uk-news/jack-nicholson-i-warned-heath-ledger -289450.
30. Greene. *Insomniac*, p. 191.
31. Foldvary-Schaefer. *The Cleveland Clinic Guide to Sleep Disorders*, p. 121.
32. John Cline. "Cognitive Behavioral Therapy for Insomnia, Part 4: Sleep Restriction." *Psychology Today*, July 13, 2009. www.psychologytoday.com/blog/sleepless-in-america /200907/cognitive-behavioral-therapy-insomnia-part-4-sleep -restriction.

Chapter Four: Adopting Good Sleep Strategies

33. University of Maryland Medical Center. "Sleep Hygiene: Healthy Hints to Help You Sleep." www.umm.edu/sleep /sleep_hyg.htm.
34. Russell Rosenberg. "How Alcohol Can Ruin Your Sleep." *Huffington Post*, August 1, 2011. www.huffingtonpost.com /russell-rosenberg-phd/alcohol-sleep_b_902578.html.
35. Greene. *Insomniac*, p. 313.
36. Julianne Taylor. "Caffeine Affects Your Sleep. No Ifs No Buts." Julianne's Paleo and Zone Nutrition, March 20, 2011. http://paleozonenutrition.com/2011/03/20/caffeine -affects-your-sleep-no-ifs-no-buts/.
37. Lisa Turner. "Sleep Advice: 5 Foods to Help You Snooze." *Huffington Post*, January 25, 2010. www.huffingtonpost .com/lisa-turner/sleep-advice-5-foods-to-h_b_430606.html.

38. Quoted in Ella Brooks. "15 Sneaky Sleep Stealers." *Natural Health*, December 2011, p. 62.

39. Quoted in Jean Enersen. "Spicy Food at Bedtime Can Disrupt Sleep." King5.com, July 21, 2010. www.king5 .com/health/Spicy-foods-may-be-keeping-you-up-at -night-98969739.html.

40. Michael Breus. "The Sleep-Weight Connection: Gender Matters." *Insomnia Blog*, November 1, 2011. www.thein somniablog.com/the_insomnia_blog/2011/11/index.html.

41. Quoted in Margarita Tartakovsky. "12 Ways to Shut Off Your Brain Before Bedtime." Psych Central. http://psy chcentral.com/lib/2011/12-ways-to-shut-off-your-brain -before-bedtime/.

42. Quoted in Tartakovsky. "12 Ways to Shut Off Your Brain Before Bedtime."

43. Michael Breus. "Sleep Vacations, Away and at Home." *Insomnia Blog*, February 28, 2012. www.theinsomniablog .com/the_insomnia_blog/page/4/.

44. Hector. Personal interview with the author. Las Cruces, New Mexico, July 18, 2012.

Chapter Five: Looking to the Future

45. Science Daily. "Gene Affecting the Ability to Sleep Discovered in Fruit Flies," February 20, 2012. www.sciencedaily .com/releases/2012/02/120220211013.htm.

46. EurekAlert. "Restless Legs Syndrome in Fruit Flies: Mutation in Fly Version of a Human RLS Gene Disturbs Sleep," May 31, 2012. www.eurekalert.org/pub_releases/2012-05 /eu-rls053012.php.

47. Quoted in Alice Park. "What Good Is Sleep? New Lessons from the Fruit Fly." *Time*, April 2, 2009. www.time.com /time/health/article/0,8599,1889099,00.html.

48. Quoted in Science Daily. "Protein Keeps Sleep-Deprived Flies Ready to Learn," May 5, 2011. www.sciencedaily.com /releases/2011/05/110505123952.htm.

49. Quoted in Jennifer O'Brien. "Sleep Apnea Linked to Increased Risk of Dementia in Elderly Women." University of California at San Francisco, August 9, 2011. www.ucsf .edu/news/2011/08/10408/sleep-apnea-linked-increased -risk-dementia-elderly-women.

50. Michael Breus. "Can Sleep Heal Painful Memories?" *Insomnia Blog*, January 26, 2012. www.theinsomniablog .com/the_insomnia_blog/2012/01/index.html.

51. Quoted in Albert Einstein College of Medicine. "Kids' Snoring Linked to Hyperactivity," March 5, 2012. www .einstein.yu.edu/news/releases/771/kids-abnormal-breath ing-during-sleep-linked-to-increased-risk-for-behavioral -difficulties/.

52. Quoted in Tara Parker-Pope. "The School Bully Is Sleepy." *Well* (blog), NYTimes.com, June 2, 2011. http://well.blogs .nytimes.com/2011/06/02/the-school-bully-is-sleepy/#more _53425.

53. Quoted in Alice Park. "Study: How Our Brains Make Us Light or Heavy Sleepers." *Time*, August 9, 2010. www .time.com/time/health/article/0,8599,2009401,00.html.

Glossary

bruxism: Teeth grinding during sleep.

cataplexy: Episodes of temporary paralysis connected to narcolepsy.

circadian rhythm: The body's biological clock that directs the timing of when the body sleeps and wakes.

cognitive ability: Ability to think, learn, and reason.

delayed sleep phase syndrome: Inability to fall asleep until late in the night or early morning with difficulty awakening until late in the morning or afternoon.

electroencephalograph (EEG): A machine that records brain waves.

homeostasis: The body's maintaining of a balanced state.

hormones: Chemicals produced by the body to trigger various functions.

hypersomnia: Sleep disorder that causes excessive sleepiness.

hypnotics: A class of drugs used to induce sleepiness.

hypocretin: A chemical released by the brain that helps regulate sleep.

insomnia: A specific sleep disorder and a symptom of other sleep disorders characterized by the inability to fall or stay asleep.

melatonin: A chemical that helps regulate sleep and waking.

narcolepsy: A sleep disorder that causes people to involuntarily fall asleep.

non-rapid-eye-movement (nREM) sleep: Three stages of sleep in which brain waves slow down and no rapid eye movement occurs.

obesity: A condition of having an abnormal amount of body fat, usually at least 20 percent above healthy weight.

parasomnia: A sleep disorder characterized by sleepers' performing involuntary physical activities of which they are unaware.

polysomnograph: A machine that records sleep patterns.

rapid-eye-movement (REM) sleep: Sleep stage characterized by rapid eye movement under closed eyelids, active brain activity, and dreaming.

restless legs syndrome: A sleep disorder characterized by a burning, tingling, or itchy feeling deep within the legs that disrupts sleep.

sleep apnea: A sleep disorder characterized by disordered breathing.

sleep debt: The difference between the amount of sleep people need and the amount of sleep they get.

sleep hygiene: Healthy sleep habits.

slow-wave sleep: Deep sleep characterized by slow brain waves, which occurs in stage three sleep.

Organizations to Contact

American Sleep Apnea Association

1424 K St. NW, Ste. 302
Washington, DC 20005
Phone: (202) 293-3650
E-mail: asaa@sleepapnea.org
Website: www.sleepapnea.org

This organization provides information about sleep apnea and
the use of positive airway pressure machines.

American Sleep Association

614 S. Eighth St., Ste. 282
Philadelphia, PA 19147
Phone: (433) 593-2285
E-mail: sleep@sleep.com
Website: www.sleepassociation.org/index.php

The American Sleep Association provides information about
sleep and sleep disorders. The website has links to recent
news articles, sleep centers, and a chat room for people with
sleep disorders.

Narcolepsy Network

129 Waterwheel Ln.
North Kingston, RI 02852
Phone: (888) 292-6522
E-mail: narnet@narcolepsynetwork.org
Website: www.narcolepsynetwork.org

The Narcolepsy Network is dedicated to helping people with
narcolepsy. It offers information about the condition, support
groups, and ongoing research.

National Sleep Foundation

1522 K St. NW, Ste. 500
Washington, DC 20005
Phone: (202) 347-3471
E-mail: natsleep@erols.com
Website: www.sleepfoundation.org

The foundation is dedicated to educating the public about the importance of sleep. It provides information on every aspect of sleep and sleep disorders. It publishes a monthly magazine called *Sleep Matters.*

For More Information

Books

Sylvia Engdahl. *Sleep Disorders*. Perspectives on Diseases and Disorders. Detroit: Greenhaven, 2011. This book consists of a series of articles on sleep disorders from various sources. Includes information about different sleep disorders, what they are, how people live with them, and controversies surrounding them.

Hal Marcovitz. *Sleep Disorders*. San Diego: ReferencePoint, 2009. This book offers a compact, well-organized overview of what sleep disorders are, their causes, and their treatment.

Mary Brophy Marcus. *Sleep Disorders*. New York: Chelsea House, 2009. This book looks at the causes, effects, and treatment of different sleep disorders.

Judy Monroe Peterson. *Frequently Asked Questions About Sleep and Sleep Deprivation*. New York: Rosen, 2010. This book provides facts about sleep and sleep deprivation in an easy-to-read question-and-answer format.

Mali Rebecca Schantz-Field. *Sleep Drugs*. New York: Chelsea House, 2011. This book looks at different sleep medications, how the drugs work, how they affect the brain and the body, and controversies surrounding them.

Periodicals

Lawrence Epstein. "The Surprising Toll of Sleep Deprivation." *Newsweek*, July 5, 2010.

Jeffrey Kluger. "SHHH! Genius at Work." *Time*, April 23, 2012.

David K. Randall. "Rethinking Sleep." *New York Times*, September 22, 2012.

Bonnie Rochman. "Please, Please Go to Sleep." *Time*, March 26, 2012.

Natalie Sylvester. "Sleep, Who Needs It? Sleep Disorders in Teens Are More Common—and More Serious—than You Think." *Current Health Teens*, November 2011.

Internet Sources

Harvard Medical School. "Healthy Sleep." http://healthysleep .med.harvard.edu/healthy/.

KidsHealth. "Common Sleep Problems." http://kidshealth.org /teen/your_body/take_care/sleep.html.

Medline Plus. "Sleep Disorders." www.nlm.nih.gov/medline plus/sleepdisorders.html.

Websites

Sleep and You Blog (www.sleepandyou.com/blog). This blog is sponsored by Sleep Health Centers, a national network of sleep centers, and authored by sleep specialists. It presents articles and information about sleep and sleep disorders.

Sleep Better (http://sleepbetter.org). Information about sleep, sleep apnea, sleep news, beds and bedding, sleep advice, plus videos can all be found on this helpful site.

Sleepnet (www.sleepnet.com). This website provides a wealth of information about sleep and sleep disorders, tips for better sleep, and links to other sleep sites.

Talk About Sleep (www.talkaboutsleep.com). This site provides sleep information and resources, including information on sleep disorders, treatment, a sleep assessment quiz, and patients' stories.

Index

Picture Credits

About the Author

Barbara Sheen is the author of more than seventy books for young people. She lives in New Mexico with her family. In her spare time, she likes to swim, walk, garden, and read. Of course, she enjoys a good night's sleep.